Accession
36013760

KT-476-655

prenatal
tests

the facts

LIBRARY
ACC. No.   DEPT.
36013760   ∩
CLASS No.
WB 320 76 DEC
WITHDRAWN
UNIVERSITY
OF CHESTER

also available in the series

prenatal
tests

the facts

LACHLAN DE CRESPIGNY
Honorary Research Fellow
Murdoch Children's Research Institute;
Obstetrician Sonologist,
Mercy Hospital for Women
Melbourne, Australia

FRANK CHERVENAK
Given Foundation Professor and Chairman
Department of Obstetrics and Gynecology
New York Weill Cornell Medical Center
New York, USA

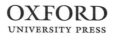

OXFORD
UNIVERSITY PRESS

OXFORD

UNIVERSITY PRESS

Great Clarendon Street, Oxford OX2 6DP

Oxford University Press is a department of the University of Oxford.
It furthers the University's objective of excellence in research, scholarship,
and education by publishing worldwide in

Oxford New York

Auckland Cape Town Dar es Salaam Hong Kong Karachi
Kuala Lumpur Madrid Melbourne Mexico City Nairobi
New Delhi Shanghai Taipei Toronto

With offices in

Argentina Austria Brazil Chile Czech Republic France Greece
Guatemala Hungary Italy Japan Poland Portugal Singapore
South Korea Switzerland Thailand Turkey Ukraine Vietnam

Oxford is a registered trade mark of Oxford University Press
in the UK and in certain other countries

Published in the United States
by Oxford University Press Inc., New York

© Oxford University Press, 2006

The moral rights of the authors have been asserted
Database right Oxford University Press (maker)

First published 2006

All rights reserved. No part of this publication may be reproduced,
stored in a retrieval system, or transmitted, in any form or by any means,
without the prior permission in writing of Oxford University Press,
or as expressly permitted by law, or under terms agreed with the appropriate
reprographics rights organization. Enquiries concerning reproduction
outside the scope of the above should be sent to the Rights Department,
Oxford University Press, at the address above

You must not circulate this book in any other binding or cover
and you must impose the same condition on any acquirer

British Library Cataloguing in Publication Data

Data available

Library of Congress Cataloging in Publication Data

Prenatal tests: the facts / Lachlan de Crespigny and Frank A. Chervenak
Includes index
1. Prenatal diagnosis—Popular works. 2. Consumer education.
I. Chervenak, Frank A. II. Title
RG628.D38 2005   618.3'2075—dc22   2005107359

Typeset by Newgen Imaging Systems (P) Ltd., Chennai, India
Printed in Great Britain
on acid-free paper by
Clays Ltd., Bungay, Suffolk

ISBN 0–19–852084–0 (Pbk.:alk.paper)   978–0–19–852084–9 (Pbk.)

10 9 8 7 6 5 4 3 2 1

acknowledgements

The authors wish to thank General Electric (who provided Figs 4.1, 7.2, and 7.11) and Philips Medical Systems who provided or assisted with production of the other ultrasound images. Lachlan de Crespigny also wishes to acknowledge Mark Pertile, Head of Prenatal Cytogenetics at Genetic Health, Victoria Australia, who kindly provided the karyotypes for Figs 2.1 and 2.3, Professor Bob Williamson, until recently Director at the Murdoch Children's Research Institute for his ongoing support, and Jon Hyett for his advice on current practice in the UK.

Whilst every effort has been made to ensure that the contents of this book are as complete, accurate and up to date as possible at the date of writing, the authors and Oxford University Press are not able to give any guarantee or assurance that such is the case. Readers are urged to take appropriately qualified medical advice in all cases. The information in this book is intended to be useful to the general reader, but should not be used as a means of self-diagnosis or for the prescription of medication.

contents

Introduction

It is amazing what little information is available about prenatal diagnosis in general pregnancy books designed for women. Prenatal diagnosis is either not included at all, or the information is very limited. Yet in most Western countries pregnant women have taken up prenatal testing with enthusiasm. Almost all women choose to have some prenatal testing, some women limit what they want to know about, and others want all the information they can possibly have on potential abnormalities.

In this book we hope to give you an understanding of the strengths and limitations of prenatal testing. It is designed to fill the information vacuum in the UK, the USA, and Australia. It follows on from the successful Australian book, *Which tests for my unborn baby? A guide to prenatal diagnosis* by Lachlan de Crespigny with Rhonda Dredge, first published in 1991 (2nd edition 1996). This new book is based on that successful formula, but includes a number of changes. These include a chapter layout based on weeks of pregnancy rather than types of prenatal test, and the addition of some wonderful new ultrasound images of a fetus at the different stages.

About the authors

Lachlan de Crespigny is an Obstetrician and Gynecologist who practices exclusively in ultrasound and related diagnostic procedures. He is in private practice and is an Honorary Fellow of the Murdoch Children's Research Institute and obstetrician sonologist at the Mercy Hospital for women. He has a long interest in research in his speciality, and has published widely in Australian and international journals. This book developed out of his successful book '*Which Tests for my unborn baby*' first published in 1991.

Frank Chervenak is Professor and Chairman of the Department of Obstetrics and Gynecology at Weill Medical College, Cornell University,

New York. He is an internationally recognized authority in ultrasound and ethics, having co-authored or co-edited 15 textbooks. He is the current president for the International Society of the Fetus as a Patient, as well as a member of many American and International societies of Maternal–Fetal medicine.

1 Why have prenatal tests?

The decision you make about prenatal testing may be one of the most important of your life. This is why it must be your decision, not your doctor's, your friend's or anybody else's. There are some abnormalities you may not wish to know about, and some prenatal tests have a risk of miscarriage. If you choose to limit testing, an abnormality that could have been detected may go unrecognized. On the other hand, choosing to have all the tests available can 'medicalize' what might otherwise been a happy and normal pregnancy.

Prenatal tests can be very informative, but they can also raise more questions than they answer. It can be difficult to find a balance between your need to know as much as possible about your baby, and the worry and uncertainty caused by some of the information you may be given.

All couples hope to have a 'perfect' baby. The sophisticated technology that is available for prenatal testing can mislead people into thinking that all abnormalities can be detected. This is far from the case. Less than half of the possible abnormalities your baby could be born with can be discovered before it is born.

Pregnancy is a normal state, not a disease. Should you let nature take its course and accept whatever child is delivered? Or should you put your already loved and nurtured unborn baby at additional risk to detect abnormalities? Nobody else can decide what tests you should have, nor can they decide the future of your pregnancy if an abnormality is detected. These decisions should be made by you, after discussions with your partner, and after consultation with your doctor or midwife.

Your choices are personal, involving your religious and moral beliefs and the desires and expectations of you and your family. Our aim is to help you become better informed, so that discussions with your doctor, your partner and others can be enhanced.

The main goal of prenatal testing is to offer choice. You can exercise three choices in relation to pregnancy testing:

1) You can choose which tests—if any—to have from the wide range of tests available

2) You can choose what information you want to be told from these tests

3) If an abnormality is found, you can choose whether you will continue with or terminate your pregnancy

Every couple should be encouraged to make their own decisions based on the available information about prenatal tests. But it takes time and effort to understand the issues involved. It might seem much easier to ask your doctor or midwife what he or she would recommend. Most health professionals are prepared to advise in this situation, but in reality they can only provide you with medical guidance. Their religious, moral, and family background, and their emotional investment in the pregnancy, differ from your own. You can accept the recommendation of your midwife or doctor, or you can research the issues yourself with their help, support and advice. This book aims to help you through the decision-making process, and relates the experiences of some couples that have already considered their options.

Some women decide not to have any tests at all, others choose a particular test, and some women accept all the tests available. It is important not to feel pressurized into having tests that you do not want. You will feel more confident in making an informed choice if you investigate what tests are available and think about how far you want to go with testing. You can choose the right prenatal tests for you if you understand the pros and cons of each test. Only after careful preparation can you be as sure as possible that you have made the right decision for you.

Ultimately it is the pregnant woman who must decide which prenatal tests, if any, to have. She is pregnant; it is she who has the tests. But both parents must live with the outcome. Working through the issues together is in the long-term interests of your relationship. Yet partners often differ in their goals and expectations. Understanding these differences and attempting to resolve them can strengthen a relationship.

Barbara, 42, said that making the decision about prenatal testing was one of the most difficult things she and her partner had had to face in their 21-year relationship. She described in great detail how they had decided on a course of action when faced with her unexpected pregnancy. Her final comment was most heartening. She believed that making their decision on testing was also one of the best things they had ever done in their relationship. They had talked the issues through in detail and come to understand each other's perspective, not just about the pregnancy but about their life together.

Some people who oppose prenatal testing claim that it is a 'search and destroy' exercise. But there is far more to it than that. There are many reasons to have prenatal testing. Some women who would not have an abortion still choose to have prenatal testing.

Advantages and disadvantages of prenatal tests

Advantages

Confidence

Prenatal test results can give some older couples, as well as those who have previously had a child with an abnormality, the confidence to try for a baby.

In Robyn's first pregnancy the vessels in the umbilical cord ran through the membranes above her cervix. This resulted in the baby having a severe haemorrhage when the membranes ruptured in labor. Robyn delivered a baby girl, Marlo, who was severely brain damaged due to the haemorrhage and who also, unexpectedly, had Down syndrome. After five days of distress and uncertainty, the baby died.

Robyn and her partner Peter were referred to counseling to discuss their options for prenatal testing. Although this was many months after Marlo had died, they both cried bitterly as they retold the story of Marlo's five days of life. They were afraid to embark on another pregnancy unless they had reassurance that the disaster of their previous experience would not be repeated. They were reassured that chorionic villus sampling (CVS) or amniocentesis would exclude a chromosomal abnormality, and that the condition which had caused the haemorrhage should be detected with ultrasound during the pregnancy. They were greatly relieved to learn that appropriate testing could prevent a repeat of the tragic experience of their last pregnancy.

Robyn and Peter went on to successfully have another child.

Reassurance

Most pregnant women get normal test results. They can then relax and enjoy their pregnancy with some uncertainties removed.

Treatment

A few conditions can be treated before the baby is born—a blood transfusion can be given for anaemia, and drugs to slow a rapid heart rate.

Preparation

If a problem is detected, couples have time to prepare themselves for the birth of their baby, and to seek information from experts and support groups. For example, if a cleft lip (harelip) has been found, there are special feeding techniques to learn.

The question that is probably the most important of all—was it better to know of Sarah's cleft lip prior to her birth? It certainly gave us time to prepare in many ways. We researched which plastic surgeons to go to, what feeding apparatus was most appropriate, and what future operations were needed. Lucy

Organization

It is safer for some babies with abnormalities to be delivered by caesarean section—knowing about this enables it to be arranged in advance.

Special care

Some babies, for example those with heart abnormalities, may need immediate specialist care and treatment. This can be on hand if abnormalities have been detected before birth.

Termination as an option

It is difficult to pre-plan how you would react if an abnormality was found. Some women who are opposed to abortion might reconsider if an abnormality is so severe that the baby was unlikely to survive after birth, other women may decide to get prepared for the particular problems their baby may have.

Disadvantages

Worry and uncertainty

The process of testing and then waiting for the results can be worrying and stressful. The results themselves can be confusing and often raise more questions than give answers.

No guarantee of perfection

You may think that a good test result guarantees a perfect baby—but in reality less than half of all abnormalities can be detected prenatally.

Risk

Some prenatal tests have risks. Amniocentesis and CVS have a small risk of miscarriage that must be weighed up against their potential benefits (see Chapters 5 and 6).

Medicalization of pregnancy

Prenatal testing can turn a happy normal experience into a medical event. This is certainly the case if a possible problem is found.

A tentative pregnancy

You may have to wait until halfway through your pregnancy for the final test results. You may not be sure you will have a baby until the test results come back normal.

Cost

Not all tests are available to all women in all health systems. The tests and good quality equipment can be expensive.

Making a decision

Some people find the issues so complex that talking to somebody outside the family, such as a health professional or a counselor is helpful. Doctors, counselors and midwives can help you weigh up the pros and cons of prenatal tests by giving you information and by helping you understand what tests best satisfy your goals.

I could not freely express my concerns to friends. Talking to a counselor allowed my to lay all my cards on the table because I knew this information would not go any further. If I had discussed the issues with friends I would be spending a lot of time explaining why I now feel so happy, apologizing for causing them concern and going over and over the ground because people are very curious.

People are well intentioned but are not trained, so the discussion may not lead to a positive outcome. In my experience people are curious and may inadvertently make a comment which plays on a person's mind. Untrained people want to interpret what they are being told by putting it into the context of their own lives. This is not helpful because their experience is unique to them. A counselor knows not to belittle the strength of an individual's feelings. A counselor is able to contribute the experiences of past clients. It can be helpful for to know you are not alone in feeling concerned.

The interview with the counselor was enormously reassuring, as up to that point I could not persuade anyone to take me seriously. They all kept telling me I was too young for a chorionic villus sampling (CVS) test or an amniocentesis—I did not fit all the guidelines. Having my feelings acknowledged gave me the confidence to proceed with the testing. If I had not done this, I believe the rest of the pregnancy would have been a nightmare and I might not have bonded with my baby. I needed the opportunity to talk through how I felt and to clarify what I needed to do to enable me to come to terms with the pregnancy. Julia

The reasoning of Penny, who at 33 had an amniocentesis for her first child, despite being regarded as low risk, illustrates the difficulty involved in imposing strict age limits on tests.

I had done a lot of work with children with intellectual disabilities and a number of their parents were quite young. Just because I was a couple of years younger than the usual testing time I didn't think that was sufficient insurance. I knew my life options would mean continuing working, and having a disabled child would make this difficult. I had thought through the issue, and I decided I was prepared to terminate the pregnancy if it was a Down syndrome fetus.

The results were normal, but unfortunately Penny's baby was stillborn. Pregnant again a year later, she once more pushed for testing, despite the trauma of having already lost a baby.

I knew it would be awful, but just because I had lost one baby didn't mean I wanted a disabled child. There was a lot of opposition from women in my support group who had also lost babies. Some were so desperate to have another child, they said: 'Give me one no matter what is wrong with it'. I still wasn't considered to be in the high-risk group and it was much harder to get a test than 12 months before. My obstetrician was supportive.

See Chapter 2 Table 5: Rising risk of Down syndrome with age.

What happens if an abnormality is found?

Many women leave decisions about prenatal testing to their midwife or doctor. But doctors are experts in medicine, they are not experts in what is right for you. This may be especially true if an abnormality is found.

Much of medicine involves advising patients what treatments are best for them. For example, if a patient presents to her doctor with abdominal pain the doctor may diagnose appendicitis. The patient would expect the doctor to advise what tests should be carried out and what the treatment should be—in this case an appendectomy operation. Appendicitis is a medical condition and thanks to the doctor's medical training he or she can advise on the best treatment. But prenatal diagnosis is quite different.

Treatments are available for only a minority of fetuses with abnormalities; a detected abnormality will not usually change how your pregnancy or labor is managed. Do you want prenatal testing if the only likely course of action is abortion if there is a problem? If an abnormality is found, who decides if the abnormality is severe enough to warrant an abortion? Only the pregnant woman can make this difficult decision. To do this she needs to be armed with as much information as possible about risks, the effect the abnormality will have on the future child's life, and the views of her partner or others who are close to her.

We all have differing views on what abnormalities, if any, are severe enough to justify abortion. These views depend on many factors including our upbringing, our approach to disability and our attitude to abortion. Surveys have shown that doctors have the same broad range of opinions on these matters as the rest of the community. Some doctors believe that abortion should be entirely the choice of a pregnant woman, whereas others believe that it should not be available to women whose fetus is diagnosed with a 'minor' abnormality such as a cleft lip and palate. Some doctors are opposed to abortion even if there is a severe abnormality. It is unlikely that your doctor or midwife will have exactly the same approach to these complex issues as you have.

Some people believe that choosing to have an abortion when an abnormality is detected shows a negative attitude towards disabled people. Others see a big difference between an attitude to a fetus and attitudes towards other people. For example, many disabled people choose to have prenatal testing for a condition they themselves have, and couples often choose to have testing for a condition their previous child was born with.

See Chapter 9, 'Decisions after prenatal testing' for a fuller exploration of your options if an abnormality is found.

2 Your fetus: normal and abnormal development

It is important to know the facts about abnormalities, because this information should form the basis of your decisions about prenatal tests. Of the 4 per cent of babies born with a problem, about half are not serious and include conditions such as a port wine stain or an extra toe. Women worry about the possibility of having a baby with an abnormality although other problems such as prematurity—one in 20 births—or having an undersize baby—one in 10 births—are more likely. 'Older' pregnant women may be particularly concerned when in fact, being older increases your chance of only a small group of abnormalities, particularly Down syndrome. Prenatal testing is an excellent way of detecting many major abnormalities, but it cannot detect them all. So, it cannot guarantee a 'perfect' newborn baby, even when a full range of tests are carried out by an expert.

What is normal development?

Before considering different types of abnormalities, we need to look at how normal development occurs (see Table 1). It is remarkable how quickly and how early the fetal structures develop. Although the fetus is too small to see many abnormalities before 11 weeks, sophisticated ultrasound technology now allows us to see many of its normal structures before it is 11 weeks old.

By 12 weeks the physical development of the fetus is complete and it is big enough for modern scanning equipment to show many of its structures, particularly if a vaginal scan is used. With careful scanning, well over half of the abnormalities that are detectable on ultrasound at 18–22 weeks can be picked at 12–13 weeks.

The sex of your fetus can be identified at 12 weeks, or sometimes earlier, using ultrasound. But this is less reliable than a later scan at 18–22 weeks.

Health professionals use the first day of the last period as the 'beginning of pregnancy'. In reality it begins 2 weeks later with the release of the

Table 1 Main stages in fetal development

Days	Crown Rump Length (cm) (CRL = top of head to tip of bottom)	Features present
0		First day of last menstrual period
14		Release of egg from ovary, conception
21		Embryo implants in the wall of the uterus
28		Eyes and ears start to form, head present
35		Arms start to form
42	0.3	Spinal canal closes around spinal cord
49	1.0	Head and body well established
56	1.6	First movements occur
63	2.4	Fingers separated but toes still united
70	3.3	Heart fully formed, human appearance with eyes, eyelids, and ears
77	4.3	Bowel returns inside abdomen
84	5.5	Urine production, sex can be identified. The fetal structures are now all developed
12– 40 weeks		The fully developed fetus now grows and the organs mature to sustain life after birth.

Source: Robinson H P and Flemming J E E, 1975 *British Journal of Obstetrics and Gynaecology* **82**, 702–10.

egg from the ovary. The last period is used for convenience because the date of ovulation is seldom known with certainty.

What is abnormal development?

Physical abnormalities, or malformations, are faults or errors in the development of a part or parts of the body. They include abnormalities that can be seen, such as a missing finger, and abnormalities of the internal organs of the body, such as the development of the heart or the brain. A malformation is different from an impairment. A malformation becomes a handicap, or impairment if it cannot be fixed and is severe enough to affect the child's quality of life. For example, a clubfoot, or turned foot, is a physical malformation that can usually be fixed after birth. There is no long-term impairment and therefore no effect on quality of life.

Intellectual disability is probably the most feared abnormality. It is estimated that about one in 200 newborn babies are severely or profoundly

Table 2 Chance of a live born baby having an abnormality (in women not having prenatal tests)

Type of abnormality	Risk of abnormality	Percentage
Chromosomal abnormality	0.6/100	0.6%
Single gene disorders	1/100	1%
Other birth defects	2/100	2%
Total (approx)	3.6/100	3.6%

intellectually disabled. Many die early, so that by the age of five, 3 to 4 children per 1000 are intellectually impaired.

After physical abnormality, the second main sort of impairment is functional—problems with the way parts of the body work. The level of disability suffered by an individual depends more on how their body functions, than on the presence of a physical abnormality. Functional problems may be either a result of a physical disability, such as spina bifida causing leg paralysis, or they can happen without any physical abnormality present.

How your body works, or your level of disability after treatment, is more important than simply having a physical abnormality. For example a missing finger might cause a child no problems, but a missing thumb, if no surgery was available, would result in your child having difficulties using their hand. Sophisticated surgery can 'create' a thumb so that the child's ultimate disability would be relatively minor.

Table 2, above, shows the risk of some of the commoner and more severe abnormalities. For a description of these conditions, see pages 20–32.

What causes abnormalities?

1. Chromosomes

Each cell in the human body normally contains 46 chromosomes. There are 22 pairs of chromosomes plus two sex chromosomes—two X chromosomes for females and an X and a Y chromosome for males. Abnormalities can occur in any of the chromosomes. The commonest and the best known chromosome abnormality is Down syndrome. This occurs when there are three of the number 21 chromosomes, instead of two.

See page 20 for more on chromosomes.

2. Genetic factors

There are many genes on each chromosome. Genes are the basic hereditary material that enables us to inherit characteristics, both good and bad, from our parents. Two well known gene disorders are cystic fibrosis and Huntington's chorea.

See page 30 for more on single gene disorders.

3. Environmental factors

Since the discovery that drugs such as thalidomide and infections such as rubella or German measles can result in abnormalities, many other external factors that can affect the developing fetus have been identified. These include:

i) Prescription drugs including anti-epileptic drugs, tetracyclines (an antibiotic) as well as thalidomide. Non-prescription drugs including alcohol, smoking, cocaine and amphetamines.

ii) Some infections including rubella (German measles), cytomegalovirus, toxoplasmosis, and parvovirus (or 'slap cheek' virus—this does not cause fetal abnormalities but can cause anaemia).

iii) Medical conditions affecting the pregnant women, including diabetes.

4. Combined factors and unknown causes

Some abnormalities arise from the combination of genetic factors and environmental factors. The cause of most birth defects is unknown.

Which abnormalities can be detected before birth?

Many women wrongly think that 'normal' prenatal test results are a stamp of normality on the fetus. But normal prenatal test results do not guarantee a 'perfect' baby. Many abnormalities are detectable, but standard testing cannot identify all abnormalities.

Screening tests are given to large numbers of women and they identify a smaller group who are at increased risk of a problem. A diagnostic test tells you for sure whether a fetus has a specific condition. Some diagnostic tests involve extra risk to the pregnancy as they involve passing a needle into the uterus to take a specimen of fluid or tissue for analysis.

Most, but not all fetuses with the physical abnormalities shown in Table 3 (following page), can now be detected by an ultrasound examination.

Table 3 Chance of some important abnormalities in live born babies

Abnormality	Number per 1000 live births
Heart abnormality	8
Kidney abnormality	8
Neural tube defects/spina bifida & anencephaly	approximately 2 (varies between countries)
Cleft (hare) lip +/− cleft palate	1.4
Club (or turned) foot	1.2
Hydrocephaly (water on the brain)	0.5–3
Abdominal wall deficiency	0.2
Dwarfism	0.2

Ultrasound is the method of detecting physical malformations; at 18–22 weeks a scan will find a significant abnormality in up to one in 100 pregnancies.

How many are found depend partly on when the ultrasound scan is carried out. For example, dwarfism or hydrocephaly may not be seen on ultrasound until after 20 weeks of pregnancy.

Many other abnormalities, such as a heart defect or clubfoot, can be diagnosed at the 12–13 week scan, although the detection rate is higher at the 18–22 week scan when the fetus is bigger. The effect of a child's heart abnormality can be known to some extent. Although there may be other unexpected abnormalities or complications, some idea of the outcome can usually be predicted.

Whether kidney abnormalities are detected depends on what the abnormality is. Some cannot be found until relatively late in pregnancy and others may not be detectable at all. Ultrasound can provide useful information on how the kidneys and bladder are functioning as the bladder normally empties urine into the amniotic fluid. Any blockage or build-up of urine in the kidneys or bladder can be seen on ultrasound.

Detection of neural tube defects (NTDs) has long been a focus of prenatal testing. This is because they are relatively common and cause severe handicap. They can now be reliably detected and preventative treatment is available in the form of folic acid supplements (see page 19). Although ultrasound is *the* method of checking fetal development, testing the level of alpha-fetoprotein (AFP) in your blood, can also suggest a physical abnormality. An increased level of AFP is found in a pregnant woman's blood in most cases of neural tube defect (spina bifida and anencephaly), and in some other abnormalities (such as omphalocele, a deficiency in the abdominal wall). For more on NTDs see page 18.

Although pictures can be obtained of the brain before birth, most children with cerebral palsy or intellectual handicap have normal brain structure on ultrasound. If an abnormality is seen in the brain on ultrasound before birth it may or may not affect your baby—unfortunately the severity of the problem is often unpredictable.

At the most, 40 per cent of intellectual disability is due to a chromosome abnormality and can be detected before birth. Down syndrome is by far the most common chromosomal condition (see page 24), followed by Fragile X syndrome, an inherited condition in which the X chromosome has an abnormality. The remaining 60 per cent of intellectually impaired babies cannot be detected before birth. Some are the result of single gene disorders (see page 30); others are the result of external factors such as infection or poorly functioning placenta. At least a third of cases have no known cause.

With current rapid advances in medical genetics, the number of abnormalities which can be diagnosed before birth is likely to increase rapidly. Prenatal diagnosis of haemophilia and cystic fibrosis has only been possible in the last few years, for example. Many uncommon or rare single gene defects can currently be detected, but there are simply too many of them for each pregnant woman to be screened for all the disorders for which tests exist. These tests are usually only available if women have a family or personal history of a particular condition, or if they are in a high risk group. An example is women who are carriers for recessive conditions such as cystic fibrosis (see single gene defects, page 31).

See Chapter 5 page 56 for details of early ultrasound and Chapter 7 page 101 for details of the mid pregnancy ultrasound scan.

Standard prenatal testing

Pregnant women are offered the following tests:

1) Ultrasound examination: a screening test that can detect many, but not all, physical abnormalities. In the best hands, ultrasound is likely to detect an abnormality in up to 1 per cent of fetuses, in particular, the more serious structural conditions.

2) Blood or serum test: a screening test that gives you an estimate of your risk of having a baby with Down syndrome or several other abnormalities.

3) Chorionic villus sampling (CVS) or amniocentesis : these are diagnostic tests which tell you for certain if your fetus has a chromosome abnormality, such as Down syndrome.

4) Additional tests and genetic counseling will be offered to women who are at special risk, such as those with a family history of a gene defect.

Interpreting the results of ultrasound screening

One of the great frustrations of ultrasound for pregnant women and their partners is that an ultrasound examination often raises more questions than it answers. There are many possible outcomes when no abnormality, or differing levels of abnormality are found on an ultrasound scan.

1. Normal result

This means that no abnormality was found, but it does not mean that there is no abnormality present. Many problems cannot be seen on ultrasound. For example, an intellectual handicap or a physical problem such as an intestinal obstruction, or a cleft palate (without a cleft lip). An abnormality might be 'missed' for technical reasons such as a difficult scan, or perhaps it was too early to detect that particular abnormality. Human error is always possible. No matter how skilled the operator is, anybody can make a mistake and miss an abnormality.

2. 'Minor' abnormalities

Many minor abnormalities can be detected with ultrasound such as a cleft lip (harelip) or a clubfoot (or turned foot). Treatment can often correct these conditions, and enable most affected children to lead full, normal, and healthy lives afterwards. When a minor abnormality is found, there is a higher chance of other abnormalities being present in a fetus. A small number of these will have other problems that were unsuspected before birth, and may result in more severe handicap.

3. Severe abnormalities

These can result in significant or profound handicap, but they are often not severe enough to cause death. One example is a hypoplastic left heart, when the left ventricle of the heart, the chamber that pumps blood to the body, is severely underdeveloped. Although operations after birth can improve the circulation, a new heart chamber cannot be surgically created, so this abnormality cannot be corrected. Operations for this condition have a high mortality rate, and the child's physical activities may be severely limited, even after several operations.

Another example is trisomy 21, or Down syndrome. This results in intellectual handicap, and physical abnormalities are common. Children with severe abnormalities have significant problems to deal with; the extent of these problems vary with the abnormality, the availability and success of treatment, the presence of associated abnormalities, and often with the intensity of education and other programmes.

4. A 'lethal' abnormality

These abnormalities are so serious that the baby cannot survive after birth. Traditionally, lethal abnormalities included anencephaly (when the bones of the skull do not form and the brain is so severely damaged that the baby usually dies before or shortly after birth), and trisomy 18 (where instead of the normal two chromosomes number 18 present there are three). Trisomy 18 usually results in multiple physical abnormalities plus profound intellectual handicap. Neonatal care is so sophisticated that there are very few newborn babies who cannot be kept alive if all available modern resources are used. Abnormalities are considered lethal if they would result in death if the baby was not treated in an intensive care unit. The uncertainty here is: will the baby really die, and if so, how long after birth?

5. Other abnormalities

Some abnormalities that are detected before birth can have a wide range of possible outcomes. Hydrocephaly, for example, may result in profound intellectual handicap and cerebral palsy, but some children born with hydrocephaly may be normal or have few problems. Similarly, a diaphragmatic hernia often causes the stomach and other abdominal organs to ride up into the chest. With treatment, the baby may survive and be perfectly healthy. Sometimes the lungs may be underdeveloped and the baby may not survive or may survive with significant respiratory problems. These uncertain outcomes create the greatest dilemma for couples. They must make a decision about whether to continue their pregnancy, knowing that the range of outcomes may vary from death, profound handicap, to living a relatively normal life. How does a couple decide what to do in this situation? Ultimately it depends on their attitude to abortion and what risks they are prepared to take.

'I just hope that we will be able to make a decision that we can both live with.' Mary

Ultrasound looks mostly for physical abnormalities, which often have an unpredictable effect on how your baby will actually function.

For early ultrasound, see Chapter 5 and for mid pregnancy ultrasound, see Chapter 7. For details on termination procedures see Chapter 9 page 135.

What are neural tube defects (NTDs)?

Neural tube defects are physical malformations of the nervous system that have a strong genetic component. Precisely how they are inherited is unknown. Your chance of having a baby with a NTD depends on a number of genes as well as external influences.

There are two main types of neural tube defect. Anencephaly is a condition where the skull and brain do not form properly, and spina bifida is when part of the spinal column is open. Babies with anencephaly are stillborn or die shortly after birth because most of the brain is missing. The problems caused by spina bifida depend on the size of the opening, its location and the amount of damage to the spinal cord and brain. If the opening is small, low in the spine, and covered by skin, there may be no problems or only mild difficulties with leg weakness and poor sensation. More often, the area is large and not covered by skin. The spinal cord and its membranes may protrude through the opening and lie in a sac on the back. This often ruptures during pregnancy or at the time of delivery. The nerves to the lower part of the baby's body, to the legs, bladder and the bowel, pass through the opening. If they are damaged, there can be some paralysis of the legs and loss of control of the bladder and bowel.

Babies with spina bifida also develop fluid on the brain (hydrocephaly) because of blockage to the flow of fluid from the brain. The baby may suffer some intellectual impairment as a result, although this may be prevented by draining excess fluid through a shunt. Children with severe spina bifida may have a short lifespan. Some have surgery to close the opening in their back. This protects against infection, but cannot give them back the abilities they have lost.

The highest rate of neural tube defects is found in Northern Ireland, where one in 120 pregnancies are affected. In Australia, the United States, and the United Kingdom, it affects about one in 500, while in Japan, less than one in 1000 are affected. If a couple has already had a baby with a NTD, or are affected themselves, the risk of subsequent pregnancies being affected rises to about one in 30. If there is a recurrence, the chances of the baby having either spina bifida or anencephaly will be equal.

Apart from women with a previously affected baby, there are some other pregnant women who have a slightly higher than normal risk of NTDs. These include couples who have a near relative with spina bifida, and women taking certain medication for epilepsy. Such women may have a risk of approximately one per cent of spina bifida being present in any pregnancy.

The incidence of NTD is not related to the age of the pregnant woman.

Can neural tube defects be prevented?

All women planning to become pregnant should know that their chance of having a baby with a neural tube defect (that is, spina bifida or anencephaly) is reduced by two thirds if they take folic acid, also known as folate supplements. Taking folate may also reduce the chance of your baby having some other abnormalities. All women planning a pregnancy should take folate supplements for at least 1 month before conception and for 6 weeks after conception. In the UK, women are advised to take it for 3 months before conception and 3 months afterwards.

If you are at low risk of spina bifida you should take 0.4 mg (400 micrograms) of folate per day. If you are at high risk you should take a supplement of 4 mg per day. Couples at high risk include those who have had a previous baby affected by a neural tube defect and women who are on medication for epilepsy. Consult your doctor or genetic counselor if you are at high risk. Folate is available over the counter at your pharmacy or health food store.

How are NTDs detected?

Ultrasound is used for diagnosing neural tube defects. After 16 weeks of pregnancy, ultrasound should diagnose about 95 per cent of fetuses with spina bifida and all those with anencephaly. A couple who have had a previous baby with spina bifida have a 1.5 per cent chance of having a baby with anencephaly and a 1.5 per cent chance of having a baby with spina bifida. If the spine and head appear normal on ultrasound, the risk of spina bifida falls to one in 1300. If the ultrasound examination is done by an experienced operator, who is able to get good views of the head and spine, an amniocentesis is not necessary. Ultrasound alone is normally used for detecting NTDs, as it will only miss spina bifida in one in 5000 births. Additional reassurance can come from a normal blood test result.

Assessing the level of a substance known as alpha-fetoprotein (AFP) in the blood and amniotic fluid was an early test developed for spina bifida. AFP is produced by the fetus prior to birth and is present in the bloodstream and spinal fluid. The level of AFP is raised in about 98 per cent of affected pregnancies. The level peaks at 13 weeks then decreases slowly until 40 weeks. If there is a defect in the skin, there will be a marked increase in the level of AFP that crosses to the amniotic fluid and into the pregnant woman's blood. AFP is one of the substances tested at mid trimester serum screening. Sometimes, the AFP level in the amniotic fluid is measured at the same time as an amniocentesis. But because spina bifida is usually seen using ultrasound, AFP is not always tested.

Another test that can also be carried out on amniotic fluid is for acetyl-cholinesterase. When levels of this enzyme are also raised, it provides extra confirmation of an abnormality. CVS cannot be used to diagnose neural tube defects.

What is a chromosome abnormality?

Each cell in our body has 46 chromosomes, arranged in 23 pairs. One of each pair is received from each parent (See Figure 2.1). The same chromosomes are present in every cell of our body. One chromosome pair, the X and Y, determine the sex of your baby. The remaining 22 pairs are called autosomes and, along with genes on the X chromosome, they determine the many characteristics of each baby, including hair and skin color, appearance, height, and intelligence. Individual chromosomes contain hundreds of genes, as shown on Figure 2.2, and each gene contains the information for one specific protein with a unique function. Each gene is located at a specific position on its chromosome and is found at the same place in all people.

About six in 1000 babies have a chromosome abnormality. Of these, around a third are due to rearrangements of chromosome material, and

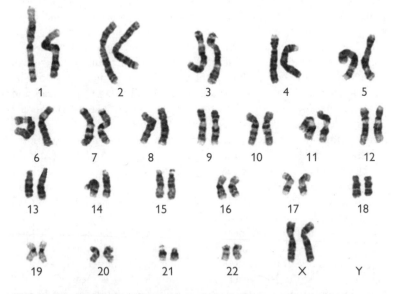

Figure 2.1 Normal chromosome analysis; in this case the chromosomes are from a female

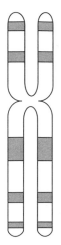

Figure 2.2 This diagram illustrates several genes in a chromosome. Each gene is located in a specific area of a specific chromosome

the rest from variations in the number of chromosomes. Table 4 on page 22 shows the more common chromosome abnormalities. Down syndrome—where there is an extra chromosome 21—is the most common, representing about half of all chromosome abnormalities in children.

'Older' pregnant women have an increased risk of a small group of chromosome abnormalities involving the autosomal trisomies. This means that instead of a chromosomal pair, there are three of a particular chromosome. The commonest autosomal trisomy is Down syndrome, called trisomy 21 because there are three of the number 21 chromosome (see Figure 2.3). The other two relatively common trisomies are trisomy 18 (Edward syndrome) and trisomy 13 (Patau syndrome). These three particular chromosome abnormalities become commoner with age. Other chromosome abnormalities and physical abnormalities tend to be relatively constant over all age groups.

If chromosome abnormality is excluded by prenatal testing then 'older' women have little increased risk of fetal abnormality.

A chromosome abnormality may be so minor that it produces no ill effects in your child, or it may be so major that it results in you having a miscarriage very early in your pregnancy. Over half of all miscarriages are associated with chromosome abnormalities, the commonest cause being triploidy, where there are three of every chromosome, resulting in a total of 69 chromosomes. There can be a range of major and minor developmental problems between these two extremes. Geneticists or experts in

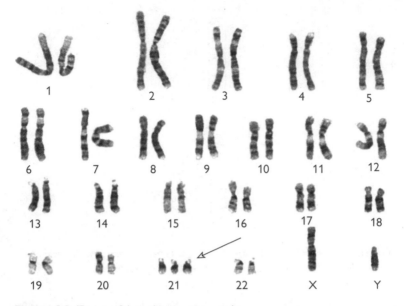

Figure 2.3 Trisomy 21, in this case in a male

Table 4 Incidence of some of the more important abnormalities in liveborn babies

Chromosome abnormality	Approx. incidence per 1000 births
Down syndrome (Trisomy 21)	1.5
XXX, XXY, XYY	1.0 each
Trisomy 18	0.3
Trisomy 13	0.3
Turner syndrome (XO)	0.2

chromosomal abnormalities can tell you what, if any, future problems might be associated with a child's particular chromosome abnormality.

About a third of chromosomal abnormalities found at birth involve variations in the number of sex chromosomes. This is where a baby has either fewer sex chromosomes than normal or has extra copies of the X or Y chromosome. While it is possible to detect these abnormalities before birth, sex chromosome variations present couples with some of the most difficult decisions because the effects may be subtle and level of disability uncertain (see page 28).

Mosaicism is a relatively common chromosomal variation found at prenatal testing. It occurs when individual cells contain different chromosomes. This person will have some features derived from each chromosomal type, and their final characteristics will depend on the relative proportions of each. A child with mosaic Down syndrome has a mixture of normal cells plus those with an extra chromosome 21. They will have some of the features of Down syndrome, but they will be less severely affected. Chromosomal mosaicism is occasionally found in the placenta during a CVS test. If this happens the baby is usually normal at birth as the chromosome mosaicism is confined to the placenta.

What are chromosomal rearrangements?

These result from breakages in the chromosomes. Sometimes, two chromosomes will have simply swapped pieces and the total amount of chromosome material will be normal. This is called a 'balanced translocation' and usually has no effect on the child. At other times, chromosome material will be lost or gained as a result of a chromosome breakage. This is called an 'unbalanced chromosome translocation' and is usually associated with intellectual impairment.

If an unbalanced translocation is found after an amniocentesis or a chorionic villus sampling (CVS) test, the baby is highly likely to have serious problems and most couples decide to terminate the pregnancy. If a balanced translocation is found, the chromosomes of the pregnant woman and her partner will be checked. Very often, one or other has the same balanced translocation, and the baby is likely to be healthy. If neither the woman nor her partner has the translocation there is a small chance that the child will have some abnormalities.

What are the tests for chromosome abnormalities?

Amniocentesis and chorionic villus sampling (CVS) are called diagnostic tests because they can give you a definite answer on whether or not your fetus has a chromosomal abnormality. Because genetic testing only tells you about the chromosomes, and not about the severity of any future disabilities, it can be quite confusing for couples considering what action to take.

The cells in your placenta and floating in your amniotic fluid come from your fetus. These cells have the same chromosomes as your fetus. Amniocentesis involves extracting an amount of amniotic fluid from around the fetus, and analyzing the cells it contains. As only a few cells are shed into the amniotic fluid, a relatively large amount of fluid—around 15 ml—needs to be taken to find enough cells for reliable chromosome analysis. (See Chapter 7 for more details of amniocentesis.)

Chorionic villus sampling (CVS) involves the analysis of cells from the developing placenta (or chorion) (see Chapter 5 for details). Fetal blood is occasionally sampled from the umbilical cord, for example, if there is doubt about the results of amniocentesis. Specimens can be taken from other parts of the fetus's body, such as urine from the bladder, but this is rarely done.

What is Down syndrome?

Down syndrome, or trisomy 21, was previously called mongolism. One in 660 newborn babies have Down syndrome. The majority of these occur 'out of the blue' to couples with no family history of chromosome abnormalities. Down syndrome has become a focus of antenatal diagnosis because it is the most frequent chromosomal abnormality resulting in a major disability in a surviving child. Many of the other chromosome abnormalities produce either minor defects, or such major ones that they result in death before or soon after birth.

Children with Down syndrome are intellectually impaired and usually have an IQ of between 25 and 50—although slightly higher scores may be achieved with early education. These children are also likely to have a number of other problems, for example, 40 per cent have a heart abnormality.

The chance of having a baby with Down syndrome increases with the age of the pregnant woman—the age of her partner has minimal influence (see Figure 2.4). All of the eggs a woman produces during her lifetime are present in a primitive stage in her ovaries when she is born. It is believed that with the passage of years, and the ageing of these eggs, there is an increased likelihood of chromosome abnormalities. While the risk of having a Down syndrome baby increases with the pregnant woman's age, not all of the extra chromosome 21s come from her. About one in 10 come from her partner.

Table 5 shows your chance of having a baby with a chromosome abnormality at any given age. The left column shows the chance of a woman delivering a live baby with Down syndrome. The next column shows the chance the same woman has of having Down syndrome detected by an amniocentesis at 16 weeks. The third column shows the chance of a fetus with any chromosomal abnormality being detected by the amniocentesis. These include both the serious ones, such as trisomy 18, and the less serious ones, such as abnormalities of the sex chromosomes. The last two

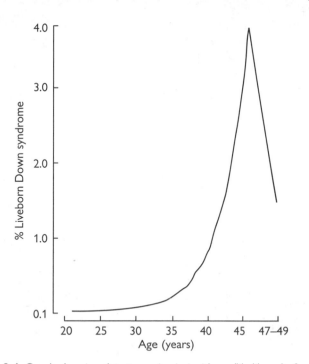

Figure 2.4 Graph showing the steep rise in incidence/likelihood of a Down syndrome baby with increasing age of the pregnant woman

columns show the chance of these conditions being present at the time of the CVS test—10 to 12 weeks. The risks are much higher in early pregnancy because fetuses with a chromosome abnormality have a high miscarriage rate. For example, one in three Down syndrome fetuses detected at 16 weeks will die before delivery.

Your risk of a Down syndrome baby

At first glance, you might think that most Down syndrome babies are born to older women, but this is not the case. Without any prenatal testing an estimated one in three (or approximately 35 per cent) of Down syndrome babies are born to women aged 35 or over. If only women over 35 years old were tested, then two-thirds of the babies with Down syndrome would not be detected. This is because most women have their babies when they are young, so even though individually they are at low risk, collectively they have more Down syndrome babies.

Table 5 Rising risk of Down syndrome with age

Age of pregnant woman	Liveborn Down syndrome[1] One in:	Amniocentesis Down syndrome[2] One in:	Amniocentesis All unbalanced chromosome abnormalities One in:	CVS Down syndrome[3] One in:	CVS All unbalanced chromosome abnormalities One in:
21	1520				
23	1450				
25	1350				
27	1200				
29	1010	These figures unavailable*			
30	890				
31	775				
32	660				
33	545	420	200		
34	445	320	160		
35	355	280	120	240	115
36	300	250	100	205	85
37	220	180	80	155	65

Age					
38	165	135	65	115	50
39	125	100	52	85	39
40	90	75	42	65	30
41	70	60	33	45	22
42	50	45	26	35	17
43	40	35	20	25	13
44			17		10
45			14		8
46			11		6
47			8		4
48			6		3
49			5		

* These figures are unavailable because these tests have been offered on a regular basis only to 'older' women.

Sources:

[1] Age 21–35: Hecht CA and Hook EB. (1994) *Prenat Diag* **14**, 729–38.
  36+ Halliday JL, Watson LF, Lumely J, et al. (1995) *Prenat Diagn* **15**, 455–65.

[2] Age 21–35: Hook EB. Prevalence, risk, and recurrence (1992). In: *Prenatal Diagnosis and Screening*, (ed.) Brock DJH, Rodeck CH, and Ferguson-Smith MA. Edinburgh: Churchill Livingstone, pp351–392.
  36+ Halliday JL, Watson LF, Lumely J, et al. (1995) *Prenat Diagn* **15**, 455–65.

[3] Hook EB. Prevalence, risk, and recurrence (1992). In: *Prenatal Diagnosis and Screening*, (ed.) Brock DJH, Rodeck CH, and Ferguson-Smith MA. Edinburgh: Churchill Livingstone, pp351–392.

If you have already had one baby with Down syndrome, then the chance of you having a second Down syndrome baby can increase. If you are under 30, the risk of a chromosome abnormality in each subsequent pregnancy is one in 100. Your risk remains the same if you are over 30. These figures are not absolute—and geneticists may use slightly different figures.

Analyzing figures on your risk is difficult. Which is the most important figure? Is it the chance of finding a Down syndrome fetus at amniocentesis or CVS, or is it your chance of giving birth to a baby with Down syndrome? The figures in Table 5 are for couples to use as they feel appropriate.

There is a rare type of Down syndrome, called translocation Down syndrome, where the abnormality can run in families. This is an uncommon problem, and affects only 3 per cent of Down syndrome babies. But it is important to test the parents of a baby with this type of Down syndrome for a particular rearrangement of chromosomes. This can put themselves and other family members at greater risk of having another baby with the syndrome.

What is trisomy 18 (Edward syndrome)?

Trisomy 18 usually causes the fetus to die during pregnancy or shortly after birth. A small percentage of these babies survive longer with profound intellectual incapacity. They often have limb and heart abnormalities, cleft lip and other physical problems.

What is trisomy 13 (Patau syndrome)?

Trisomy 13 has a similar outcome and intellectual problems as trisomy 18. Major abnormalities of the brain, face and heart are common.

What are sex chromosome variations?

About a third of chromosome abnormalities are sex chromosome variations. These present couples with some of the most difficult decisions because the abnormalities may be subtle and the level of disability may be uncertain.

Until the mid 1960s, knowledge about people with sex chromosome anomalies was based entirely on those who showed clinical symptoms, particularly intellectual impairment and behavioural problems. This provided a false view of sex chromosome abnormalities because the most severely affected people were used to define the problems. Since then, large-scale screening of newborn infants has shown that one in 400 newborns has a sex chromosome variation, and we now know that most of these will live relatively normal lives.

Newborn chromosome surveys began in the mid 1960s and continued over the next decade. They aimed to find out what kind of effect sex chromosome variations had on development. Some 307 children were identified and followed up in seven studies of consecutive live births in the United States, Canada, Denmark and Scotland. Girls with an extra X chromosome and boys with either an extra Y or X were found to be the most common, each with an incidence each of one in every 1000 births.

Girls with an extra X chromosome (47XXX) are taller than average and may have delayed puberty. Two-thirds have normal intelligence, while a third have borderline IQ or intellectual impairment. Boys with an extra X chromosome (47XXY), known as Kleinfelter syndrome, are also tall. They have a mild reduction in intelligence but have frequent specific learning problems. They are infertile and have delayed or incomplete puberty, which may be treated with hormones.

Boys with an extra Y chromosome (XYY syndrome) tend to be taller, are fertile, have normal intelligence and usually normal behaviour. When this condition was first discovered, a higher incidence was found among prison inmates. This led to a view that an extra Y chromosome predisposed carriers to aggressive and psychotic behaviour. However, follow-up studies have shown quite normal development in most boys with this condition, and the risk of behaviour problems seems to be lower than was first supposed.

The experiences of one couple, where an amniocentesis showed that their boy had Kleinfelter syndrome, illustrates the dilemma of couples considering the range of possible outcomes for their baby.

The outlook with Kleinfelter syndrome was not certain. Ben might simply be a tall, overweight, infertile person experiencing learning difficulties during middle childhood. Or he could be more severely intellectually disabled. He might experience puberty only with the use of continued doses of hormones. But he might not. The literature suggested that he might have a predisposition to cancers of the testes or breasts. But it might not materialize. There was evidence of predisposition to psychotic illness. But he might be lucky. The information shifted and changed depending on what we read, the research methodology and who we spoke to.

What is Turner syndrome?

Turner syndrome is a less common condition when a girl has a missing X chromosome. The resultant sex chromosome pattern is called 45X.

Turner syndrome occurs in about one in 5000 newborns. It is much commoner in early pregnancy, but most miscarry. Newborn babies with Turner syndrome may have webbing of the neck and an increased likelihood of heart and kidney abnormalities. Their intelligence is usually normal, but they may have some specific learning disabilities. These girls are of small stature and do not have functioning ovaries, so they cannot have children, except by using a donated ovum and in vitro fertilization technology.

Most fetuses with Turner syndrome can be identified with ultrasound prior to birth. Signs may include swelling of the tissues around the neck, fluid collection in other tissues, reduced amniotic fluid and poor growth. Severely affected fetuses are very unlikely to survive until birth. When a fetus is less severely affected it may survive, for example if it has minor swelling around the neck which subsides during pregnancy. If these features are detected with ultrasound, it is usual to check the fetal chromosomes. Only some will have Turner syndrome, others will either have normal chromosomes or some other abnormality.

If you are found to be carrying a fetus with a sex chromosome variation, you should see a genetic counselor. He or she will have the latest information on the condition. About half the couples presented with this finding decide to terminate the pregnancy. Your decision will be based on your own family circumstances and expectations.

What are single gene disorders?

Humans have approximately 20,000 to 25,000 genes contained within the 23 pairs of chromosomes. A gene is usually present as two copies—one copy is found on each of a particular pair of chromosomes and each parent contributes one chromosome per chromosome pair (An exception to this is the small number of genes present only on the Y sex chromosome that is found just in males.)

There are about 5,000 recognized single gene defects; most are very rare conditions, inherited from generation to generation. In the past, it has been difficult to diagnose these conditions before birth, even if a couple had a previously affected child, because one specific gene may be at fault. Some of these conditions produce an abnormal substance in the amniotic fluid or fetal blood—these conditions were the first to be diagnosed before birth.

A recent major development in diagnosis is by direct analysis of DNA, the 'building blocks' of chromosomes. Scientists throughout the world are now attempting to determine the actual site on the chromosome where each of the genes occur. As this knowledge increases, some diseases which occur because of abnormalities in either one or small numbers of genes, can be diagnosed by studying the chromosome itself.

Normal genes and gene defects may be dominant or recessive. For dominant conditions, such as Huntington's disease, carriers of one copy of the gene defect will develop the disease. An affected parent will then have a one in two chance of passing it on to each of his or her children. Recessive conditions like cystic fibrosis are more common and quite harmless to those who carry only one copy of the gene. For the disease to manifest, both parents must be carriers of the gene defect. The risk to each of their children is then one in four.

While many single gene disorders produce seriously debilitating illnesses, they are also very rare, and their frequency varies between geographic regions. Prenatal testing for couples with a family history or an affected child can give vital support and help. This can give some couples the courage to have a family. A genetic counselor will be able to tell you the chance of a defective gene being passed on to your baby and whether it is likely to cause any major problems. This is because gene defects follow clearly defined patterns of inheritance, first outlined in the nineteenth century by an Austrian monk, Gregor Mendel.

This type of prenatal analysis will only be done if there is a history of a gene disorder in the family, or if the couple already has an affected child. Some of the more common genetic diseases that can be diagnosed before birth are described below.

Cystic fibrosis

This is the most common single gene disorder in North European people, affecting about one in 2000 babies. People with cystic fibrosis have recurrent respiratory infections and may die in early adulthood. One in 20 people carry the recessive gene for cystic fibrosis, without any sign of the condition. Cystic fibrosis can be detected by the presence of abnormal enzymes in the amniotic fluid, but the results of this test can be borderline. Gene probes have now been developed which can give pregnant women at risk of this disorder a definitive result at the time of their CVS test (see Chapter 5, page 63). Population screening where everyone is tested is being considered in some countries in order to identify those couples most at risk.

Thalassaemia

This is a disorder of the red blood cells which causes major health problems in Italy, Greece, some Mediterranean islands, and parts of South-East Asia. Gene probes can be used to test most at risk pregnant women for thalassaemia. For the rest, a blood test at 18 weeks can determine whether the fetus has inherited the gene defect from both parents. One copy of the gene has little impact, while two copies result in severe anaemia and a shortened lifespan.

Huntington's disease

This causes severe body movements plus intellectual deterioration after the age of 40. If you have relatives with this disease you can be tested to find out if you will also develop it. The condition can also be diagnosed prenatally from a CVS specimen.

Haemophilia and Duchenne muscular dystrophy

These are recessive gene disorders on the X chromosome, which are only likely to affect sons of women who are carriers. Each son will have a one in two chance of being born with the disease. Haemophilia is a bleeding disorder caused by the blood lacking a clotting factor. Usually couples with a high risk of a baby with haemophilia will be tested by CVS, but some require fetal blood sampling at 18 weeks (see Chapter 7).

Duchenne muscular dystrophy results in increasing muscular weakness. It begins in early childhood and those affected usually die in early adulthood. This may also be diagnosed using chorionic villus sampling (see Chapter 5).

3 Choosing the best prenatal tests for you: an overview

You can decide not to have any prenatal tests, to have some of the tests on offer, or to have all the available tests. What you decide about prenatal testing will depend on your attitude to abnormalities and your feelings about terminating your pregnancy. When you are considering which tests are best for you, it is important to be aware of which risk factors, if any, apply in your situation. Risk factors can include your age, your pregnancy history and your health.

See Chapter 3 for risks of abnormalities generally and Chapter 6 for your risk of Down syndrome.

Diagnostic tests such as an amniocentesis and chorionic villus sampling (CVS) can tell you if your fetus has chromosomal abnormalities, but they are invasive and have a risk of miscarriage. Screening tests such as ultrasound and blood tests can detect physical abnormalities and give a risk figure for Down syndrome, but they cannot give a definitive answer on whether your fetus has a chromosome abnormality.

Summary of standard prenatal tests for abnormalities

(i) Physical or structural abnormalities
An ultrasound examination, or scan, usually in the middle stages of pregnancy, can detect physical defects such as spina bifida, missing limbs or fingers, and abnormalities of internal organs such as the heart, kidneys, and brain.

(ii) Chromosome abnormalities
There are two types of tests available for detecting chromosome abnormalities, of which Down syndrome is the commonest and most important:

Screening tests show you the level of risk of your fetus having a chromosome abnormality. Screening tests include blood tests—called 'maternal serum screening'—and an ultrasound examination at 11½–13 weeks, or a combination of the two. Ultrasound at 18–22 weeks can also show signs of Down syndrome.

Diagnostic tests tell you for certain if there is a chromosome abnormality. Those available to you are amniocentesis (see Chapter 6, page 87) or chorionic villus sampling (CVS, see Chapter 5, page 63). Diagnostic tests are options for women of any age who are particularly concerned about chromosomal abnormalities, but few women under 35 years old request them unless an increased risk is found on a screening test.

(iii) Other genetic abnormalities

There are tests available for those few couples who are at risk of having a baby with a particular abnormality; they may already have had an affected baby, or they may have a family history of genetic disease. These abnormalities include hundreds of inherited conditions including fragile X (a form of intellectual impairment), cystic fibrosis, and thalassemia.

Tests for physical or structural abnormalities

Early ultrasound examination

With good ultrasound equipment and a vaginal ultrasound transducer— a transducer is the piece of equipment that emits the sound waves—all the physical structures of the fetus that are examined in a later scan can often be seen from around 12–13 weeks. This early scan cannot replace the traditional mid pregnancy scan at 18–22 weeks. Detecting abnormalities at this time is more difficult and sometimes impossible, because the fetus is much smaller (see Chapter 5, page 55 for details of early scans).

Ultrasound at 18–22 weeks

An ultrasound examination at this time allows accurate assessment of the age of the pregnancy, the site of the placenta, whether or not you have a multiple pregnancy and checks for many structural abnormalities. (See Chapter 7, page 101 for details.) A scan at 18–22 weeks is the traditional, and still the best, time to check your fetus for structural abnormalities. It is big enough to see the physical structures well, and abortion is still available in most areas. This later scan will detect some abnormalities such as some heart problems and hydrocephaly, or water on the brain, which do not develop until after 13 weeks of pregnancy.

Serum screening at 15–18 weeks

This blood test looks for signs of neural tube defects as well as for Down syndrome. The levels of one of the substances tested, alpha-fetoprotein (AFP), is increased in the pregnant woman's blood in about 90 per cent of anencephalic pregnancies and 85 per cent of spina bifida pregnancies. A raised AFP indicates that there is an increased risk, but most women with an increased AFP level will deliver a normal, healthy baby. In America, a serum AFP test is routinely offered in the second trimester—not only to screen for anomalies but also to check for placental dysfunction. AFP levels may also be tested in the amniotic fluid taken during amniocentesis, but this is now seldom used because the diagnosis of NTDs with ultrasound is so accurate. See Chapter 6, page 83 for full details of serum screening at 15–18 weeks.

Tests for chromosome abnormalities

Prenatal tests for chromosome abnormalities, such as Down syndrome, fit into one of two categories. Those able to detect all affected fetuses are called diagnostic tests, and those able to detect only some are called screening tests. Down syndrome is usually the focus of testing because it is the most common chromosome abnormality, and the most common cause of intellectual impairment.

Diagnostic tests

There are two tests available that will diagnose virtually all cases of chromosome abnormality, including Down syndrome. These are amniocentesis, usually carried out from 15 weeks (see Chapter 6, page 87 for details); and chorionic villus sampling (CVS), carried out any time after 10 weeks of pregnancy (see Chapter 5, page 63). Both these diagnostic tests carry a small risk of miscarriage. Amniocentesis has a miscarriage rate of up to one in 200. The risk of miscarriage with CVS is thought to be slightly higher.

Screening tests

The screening tests that detect some fetuses with Down syndrome are ultrasound at 11½–13 weeks, ultrasound at 18–22 weeks, and maternal serum screening.

Ultrasound

An early ultrasound scan detects more cases of Down syndrome than a later scan. This is because six out of ten fetuses with Down syndrome have a thick layer of fluid beneath the skin at the back of their neck at 11½–13 weeks. This is called nuchal translucency. By 15 weeks this fluid will usually have been absorbed. An ultrasound examination at 18–22 weeks can identify suspicious signs or 'markers' of Down syndrome. It can also detect a range of other abnormalities not evident in earlier scans (see Chapter 7, page 119).

Serum screening tests

There are two types of serum screening, or blood tests. One is done early and one is done later in pregnancy.

a) Early serum test: Blood is taken at 9–12 weeks. Usually two substances are measured and a risk figure for Down syndrome is calculated after incorporating the age of the pregnant woman and the nuchal translucency thickness. The blood test is not accurate enough to use without including the nuchal translucency as well.

b) Later serum test: Blood is taken at 15–18 weeks and two, three, or more substances are measured. The risk of Down syndrome is calculated after incorporating the age of the woman. If the result shows that the risk of Down syndrome is higher than one in 250, an amniocentesis is offered. This late blood test detects approximately 70 per cent of Down syndrome fetuses, although results vary depending on what the laboratory measures and whether the dates are first checked with ultrasound.

The results of serum screening are better when laboratories are dealing with large numbers of specimens and they have a lot of experience.

Other genetic abnormalities

If you have already had a baby with an abnormality you may be worried about it happening again. If the abnormality was physical, an ultrasound examination at around 13 weeks may give an early diagnosis, but the scan at 18–22 weeks can detect some conditions more easily as the fetus is bigger. Couples with concerns or with a family history of specific abnormalities should discuss them with their doctor, who may refer them to a genetic counselor if the problem is complex. See Chapter 2 and Chapter 7 for details of abnormalities.

A simple guide to prenatal tests

Do you want to check the chromosomes of your fetus? If so you can choose a diagnostic or a screening test.

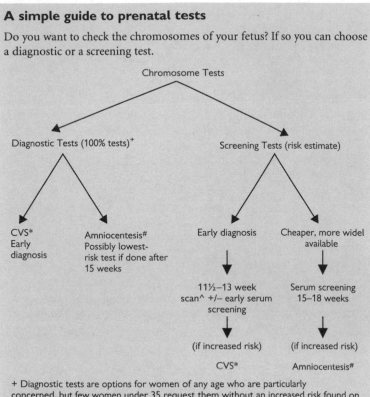

+ Diagnostic tests are options for women of any age who are particularly concerned, but few women under 35 request them without an increased risk found on ultrasound and/or serum screening (see Chapter 6).

* Termination of pregnancy performed by simple curette.

Termination of pregnancy mostly performed by induced labor.

^ In some centers an 11½–13 week scan is offered and no results are given.

Serum screening is done at 15–18 weeks and the results combined to produce a risk figure.

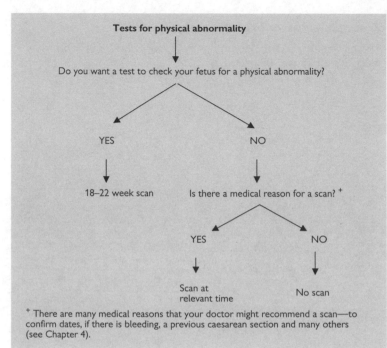

Tests for physical abnormality

Do you want a test to check your fetus for a physical abnormality?

YES   NO

18–22 week scan   Is there a medical reason for a scan? [+]

YES   NO

Scan at relevant time   No scan

[+] There are many medical reasons that your doctor might recommend a scan—to confirm dates, if there is bleeding, a previous caesarean section and many others (see Chapter 4).

4 Prenatal testing: preconception to 9 weeks

Prenatal tests are usually offered after 9 weeks. Before this, it is too early to test for abnormalities. Ultrasound scans are not usually done in the first 2 months of pregnancy, except for complications, such as bleeding or pain. An early scan can very accurately determine the age of your pregnancy—this can be important when planning prenatal tests.

What can I do before I conceive?

Think about prenatal testing

You and your partner may wish to explore your feelings about it before you become pregnant, rather than to discover you have major differences afterwards.

Arrange a pre-pregnancy check

This could be with your doctor, or midwife. It can be helpful to meet the person who will care for you in pregnancy, to ensure he or she is somebody who you can readily relate to. It can be useful to know their approach to prenatal testing and the range of tests that will be available to you. When you are pregnant, you can explore issues such as where to have your baby and attitudes to caesarean section.

Discuss pre-conception tests

There are many tests available to you before you conceive to help minimise the risks of pregnancy. Discuss the following with your health professional:

- Rubella (German measles) and varicella (chicken pox). If you are not already immune, vaccinations are available.
- Syphilis screening. This is a routine blood test.

- Screening for cystic fibrosis—this is available in some centers. Also, thalassemia screening for couples with a Mediterranean background, and Tay–Sachs screening for Ashkenazi Jews.

Take folic acid

If you take folic acid before conception, the risk of your baby having a neural tube defect such as spina bifida or anencephaly is reduced. The American College of Medical Genetics advises women to supplement their diet with 0.4 mg per day of folic acid throughout their reproductive years. If you have a previous history of neural tube defects you should have genetic counseling to discuss your risk of having an affected baby, the management of subsequent pregnancies, and the amount of folic acid you should be taking.

What does the fetus look like at 0–9 weeks?

0–3 weeks

Pregnancy is usually counted from the first day of the last menstrual period simply because it is a date that most women remember. Few women know the exact date of conception. Conception usually happens around two weeks before an expected period—around day 14 for women with a 28 day cycle. The first sign of pregnancy is usually a missed period, although sensitive pregnancy tests can be positive before this.

4–5 weeks

A tiny pregnancy sac can be seen on ultrasound when it is about a millimetre in diameter at 4½ weeks (2½ weeks after conception). It is easier to see by 5 weeks. The fetus and its heartbeat can be seen just before 6 weeks. If a scan is done earlier it is unusual to see see either the fetus or its heartbeat.

6–9 weeks

At 6 weeks the fetus can be seen inside the pregnancy sac. It is 2 mm long and looks like a dot with a moving bit in the middle. This is the heart beating at approximately 90 beats per minute. The fetus starts to take some form by 8 weeks, when it measures 1½ cm. See Figure 4.1. By 9 weeks it is 2.3 cm long and an outline of the head, body and limbs can be seen on ultrasound. See Figures 4.2 and 4.3. Some of the internal organs can also start to be seen.

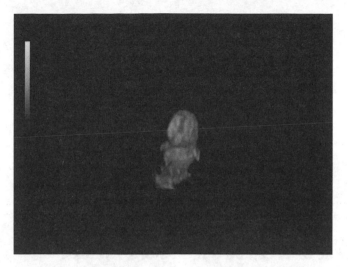

Figure 4.1 This 3D image shows that sometimes some fetal form can be identified at even this early stage (7½ weeks) with the image showing the head and the limb buds

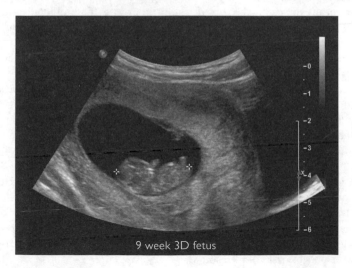

9 week 3D fetus

Figure 4.2 9 week 3D fetus

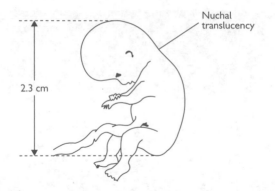

Nuchal
translucency

2.3 cm

Figure 4.3 Diagram of 9 week fetus

What tests can be done before 9 weeks?

By the time you are 9 weeks pregnant you should have met your doctor or midwife, or attended your hospital clinic, and discussed your prenatal test options. Some tests can be done as early as 10 weeks. Starting early gets some of the tests out of the way, enabling you to enjoy your pregnancy. It also means you can make your decisions in private. If a problem is found and you choose to have an abortion, this can happen before you announce your pregnancy. Don't panic if you are 10 weeks pregnant and have not yet thought about tests—the same or alternative tests can be done later in pregnancy.

Very few abnormalities can be detected with ultrasound before 10 weeks, and it is too early for chorionic villus sampling (CVS) and other tests. A scan may be offered if there are complications such as bleeding, to find out how pregnant you are, or to see if you have conceived twins (see page 46). A multiple pregnancy can be detected at 6 weeks.

Ultrasound in early pregnancy is considered safe, but the fetus is sensitive to external agents, especially in the first 3 months of pregnancy. It is recommended that scans in early pregnancy are done for medical reasons only. Higher power levels, such as Doppler, are not normally used at this time. See Chapters 5 and 7 for a full description of the early and mid pregnancy ultrasound examinations and Chapter 7 page 107 for information on the possible risks of ultrasound.

You will be given a pelvic examination or a simple abdominal palpation at this early stage and at subsequent appointments. This is when your doctor or midwife feels the overall size of your uterus by pressing down on your lower abdomen. This examination may be inaccurate as uterine size varies between women. The size of your placenta and the amount of amniotic fluid around the fetus also varies. If there is a fibroid, an ovarian cyst, or some urine in your bladder, the uterus can feel bigger than it really is.

New tests at this early stage of pregnancy will probably become available in the future. Fetal cells can be found in the blood or in a smear from the cervix of pregnant women, and researchers are hoping to develop a no-risk chromosome test using such non-invasive techniques.

How does ultrasound measure the age of my pregnancy?

An ultrasound scan works out the age of a pregnancy by measuring parts of the fetus. The earlier a scan is performed, the more accurate is the age it will give you. This is because all fetuses grow at the same rate in the first few months of pregnancy, regardless of race, size of parents or the eventual size of the baby.

The 'crown–rump length' (CRL) of the fetus (see Figure 4.4) is the measurement taken up to 13 weeks. This is a measurement taken from the top of the head to the tip of the bottom. If the fetus is too small for such details

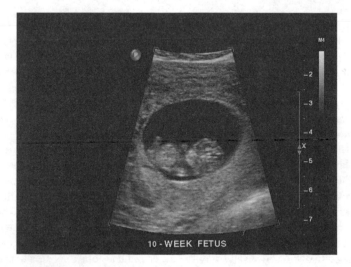

Figure 4.4 The image used to measure the crown–rump length of the fetus to assess gestation. The measurement is taken from the top of the fetal head to the tip of the bottom

to be seen, then the longest measurable length is taken to be the crown–rump length. After 13 weeks the measurements of the head and thigh bone (femur) are used.

7–10 weeks is the best time for calculating the date of conception by ultrasound—it gives a due date with an accuracy of a few days. By 13–20 weeks this accuracy is reduced to within one week either way. The nearer you get to your due date, the less accurate ultrasound becomes. In the second half of pregnancy there are large variations in growth rates. Normal birth weights at 40 weeks vary from about 2.9 kg to 4.0 kg or more. Ultrasound is very inaccurate in the last few weeks of pregnancy—estimated due dates may be as much as 3 or 4 weeks out.

Scans before 10 weeks of pregnancy are not offered routinely. You will only be offered ultrasound before 10 weeks of pregnancy if there are complications.

Why is the age of my pregnancy important?

Knowing the age of your pregnancy can help doctors treat any complications that might arise. Knowing the exact date of conception, and what stage the fetus is at, can also be important if you were exposed to a potentially dangerous substance or medication before you knew you were pregnant.

Before ultrasound scans, it was not possible for a doctor to be sure whether a small baby in late pregnancy was the result of incorrect dates or inadequate growth. Because of this uncertainty, a number of women were confined to hospital, often for many weeks. This problem has been solved by the widespread use of ultrasound in the first half of pregnancy which determines the age of your pregnancy. If you are sure when your last period began, and the size of your uterus at a pelvic examination feels right for these dates, you are likely to be fairly accurate.

Ultrasound cannot tell you when you will deliver your baby, but rather, by knowing when conception occurred, when it is due. You may deliver well before the expected date or after it. There is no way, with ultrasound or any other method, of predicting when your labor will actually begin.

Knowing your menstrual cycle can help avoid confusion about when you conceived. But nature can fool you. You may feel sure of the date of your last period, when you ovulated or when you conceived. But, it could happen that you conceived a month earlier and had some bleeding in early pregnancy which was similar to your period. Also, women often do not ovulate exactly 2 weeks after the last menstrual period, and this complicates the calculation of the due date.

LIBRARY, UNIVERSITY OF CHESTER

What is a miscarriage?

A miscarriage is the loss of a pregnancy before 20 weeks. Although miscarriage is common, most couples find it extremely upsetting and many have similar feelings of grief to those who lose a child after birth.

About 1 in 7 pregnancies end in miscarriage, but many more miscarry before the pregnancy is even recognized—the conception simply comes away with the period.

If the fetus grows for at least the first 6 weeks and then dies it can be seen on ultrasound. Doctors may call this a 'missed abortion' or 'missed miscarriage', because it has died and your body has not yet expelled it. If the fetus dies earlier than this and is too small to see on ultrasound, it is called a 'blighted ovum', or a pregnancy without a visible fetus, see Figure 4.5.

Although a fetus can die any stage of pregnancy, death is most common in the first 8 weeks. The miscarriage itself may not happen until much later, even as late as 20 weeks. In the meantime you may still feel pregnant, as the placenta continues to function and produce pregnancy hormones.

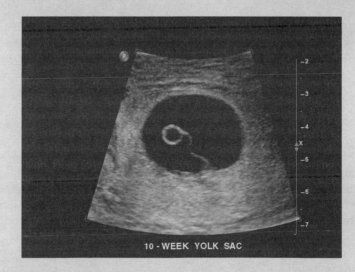

10 - WEEK YOLK SAC

Figure 4.5 An embryonic pregnancy. In the pregnancy the round circle is the yolk sac that provides early fetal nutrition but there is no demonstrable fetus. This pregnancy is also known as a blighted ovum and will end in miscarriage

There are few outward signs when a fetus dies. Your doctor may find that your uterus is smaller then expected during a routine examination, or you may notice you are not feeling so nauseous. But there could be other reasons for these changes. Occasionally a woman finds on a routine ultrasound scan that the fetus has been dead for some time and nobody had suspected it.

If you have a scan before you are 6 weeks pregnant, it is impossible to know whether the heartbeat cannot be seen because it is too early or because the fetus is dead. Another scan one week later may be needed to be sure. Whether or not you have to wait longer to get a definite answer on ultrasound depends on the experience of the person performing the ultrasound and whether or not they use a vaginal scanner.

You may not find out why your fetus died. Many deaths in early pregnancy occur because the fetus had an abnormality, particularly of the chromosomes. For your own peace of mind you should recognize that it was not because of anything you did or did not do; and that you could not have prevented it happening. After one miscarriage, the risk of miscarrying your next pregnancy is not increased.

Many people want to know the sex of the fetus they have lost. This can be difficult as death often occurs very early in pregnancy, and the sex cannot be seen on ultrasound at this time.

See page 48, 'Bleeding in pregnancy'.

Why might I be offered an ultrasound scan before 10 weeks?

Multiple pregnancy

Approximately one in 80 women who become pregnant without fertility treatment conceive twins, and one pregnancy in 6,400 are triplets. The proportion of multiple pregnancies is much higher after most infertility treatments. Ultrasound can identify the number of fetuses present from 6 weeks into the pregnancy. Twins are rarely missed on ultrasound. As a scan provides a section or a slice all the way through the pregnancy, the fetuses cannot hide behind one another.

From 6 weeks each fetus and their heartbeat become visible in each individual pregnancy sac. The number of fetuses seen is likely to be the number that you take home. Occasionally, one dies. In a multiple pregnancy the dead fetus does not miscarry, like a single fetus does. The dead fetus stays inside the uterus and eventually both deliver together. Without ultrasound, a pregnant woman would not be able to tell that a twin had died, as the healthy fetus usually keeps growing normally, the placenta still operates, and there is no bleeding.

Approximately seven in 10 twins are non-identical—coming from two separate eggs fertilized by two different sperm. Three in 10 are identical—coming from one egg, which separates into two—very early in development. The risk of complications with a twin pregnancy does not depend on whether they are identical or not, but on the placental circulations.

Twins are monochorionic if there is a single placenta with a mixing of the circulations of the two fetuses in the placenta. Monochorionic twins are always identical. Two thirds of identical twins have monochorionic placentas. Twin pregnancies that are monochorionic have a much higher rate of complications than those that are dichorionic.

Twins are dichorionic if there are two separate functioning placentas—the two placentas may be joined but there are no shared blood vessels between the two fetuses. All non-identical twins and about a third of identical twins are dichorionic.

There are increased risks with monochorionic twins because one can be getting too much blood from the placenta and the other too little. This complication is called twin to twin transfusion. This is potentially very serious, and may require premature delivery. Treatments are available but the risk of death and disability are high. These treatments include amnioreduction (drainage of excess fluid that builds up in one sac) and laser of the communicating vessels, which are discussed in Chapter 8.

In any multiple pregnancy, one fetus may die and this causes no immediate harm to the surviving fetus or fetuses, except in monochorionic multiple pregnancies. Here, when one fetus dies, its blood pressure drops, so that blood from the placenta preferentially goes to the dead fetus. The survivor receives far too little blood and may also die or be severely damaged. Because of this, monochorionic twins are monitored more intensively than dichorionic twins.

A small proportion of identical twins, about one in 100, share the same amniotic sac—they are called monoamniotic. The two umbilical cords can become tangled, causing circulation problems to one or other of the fetuses, especially in labor. Monoamniotic twins with the cords entwined are delivered by caesarean section to stop the risk of the intertwined cords tightening and obstructing during delivery.

Conjoined twins are very rare—approximately one in 50,000 live births or one in 600 twin pregnancies. The possibility of conjoined twins can be excluded once a membrane has been identified between the individual fetuses.

Bleeding in early pregnancy

Some pregnant women have bleeding in early pregnancy even though the fetus is healthy and growing normally. About one in seven women who know they are pregnant, miscarry. If you are going to miscarry, bleeding is almost always the first sign. Your risk of miscarriage is lower the less bleeding you have and the later in pregnancy you have it.

If you have bleeding in early pregnancy, your doctor may arrange an ultrasound examination for you. Ultrasound is the only test that can tell you whether your fetus is alive in early pregnancy. A pregnancy test will be positive if there is any placental tissue present; it cannot tell you about the well-being of the fetus itself.

If the fetus is alive, with its heartbeat visible, there is about an 85 per cent chance that your pregnancy will continue normally. There is no increased chance of your fetus having an abnormality. The blood is lost from you, not from the fetus.

If you have had bleeding, but your fetus has not died, your doctor or midwife will check for the following signs, which may affect your risk of a miscarriage later on in this pregnancy:

1) Fluid around the fetus—a reduced amount of fluid around the fetus in the pregnancy sac increases your chance of miscarrying. If the pregnancy continues, this fluid will slowly increase.

2) Blood clot—a small amount of blood has no effect on the developing fetus, but if the scan shows a large blood clot, there is an increased chance that you will miscarry.

3) Slow fetal heartbeat or slow rate of growth—this can be a sign of a failing pregnancy.

If the fetus has died, bleeding often continues for some weeks unless some action is taken. For this reason, many women have their uterus emptied surgically. This is called a suction curettage or a dilation and curettage (D&C). See Chapter 9 for a full description of this procedure.

Pain in early pregnancy

Pain in pregnancy, without bleeding, is very common and usually has no serious cause. It is rarely the first sign of a miscarriage. When miscarriage occurs heavy bleeding is followed by pain as the uterus contracts.

There are three important conditions that can cause pelvic pain early on and can be diagnosed using ultrasound. These are an ectopic pregnancy, ovarian cysts, and fibroids. Even if you have no other symptoms, your doctor may suspect these conditions if they feel a lump other than the pregnant uterus during an examination.

Ectopic pregnancy

An ectopic pregnancy develops outside the uterine cavity, most often inside the fallopian tube (see Figure 4.6). It can be serious, even life-threatening, as an ectopic pregnancy may rupture and bleed internally. There are occasional reports of a pregnancy in the abdomen resulting in a healthy baby, but this is very rare. Because of the dangers, treatment is considered as soon as an ectopic pregnancy is diagnosed.

Your doctor may suspect an ectopic pregnancy if you develop pain in early pregnancy or if you are at special risk. Perhaps you have had a previous ectopic pregnancy, a pelvic infection, an operation on the fallopian tubes, or infertility.

Diagnosing an ectopic pregnancy is much easier than it used to be, because of modern ultrasound equipment. A vaginal scanner can be used to locate the ectopic pregnancy outside the uterus. Or, an ectopic pregnancy can also be diagnosed if there is no visible pregnancy inside her uterus, but the woman is known to be pregnant. You may need surgery to

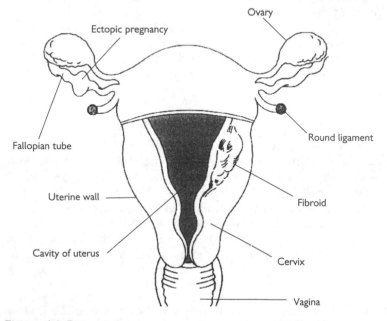

Figure 4.6 Diagram showing an ectopic pregnancy and a fibroid

confirm the diagnosis, usually a laparoscopy—an examination of the inside of the abdomen with a medical telescope.

Ultrasound cannot exclude the possibility of an ectopic pregnancy; even if there is a healthy pregnancy inside the uterus you could also have an ectopic pregnancy, but this is extremely rare. Alternatively, no matter how good the scanning equipment and the operator are, a small ectopic pregnancy could be present but not picked up on the scan. With modern equipment this is happening less often.

Ovarian cysts

Every pregnant woman has an ovarian cyst, known as the corpus luteum, in early pregnancy. It forms in the ovary after the release of the egg. Usually thin-walled, the cyst is full of fluid or blood and produces the hormones that maintain the early pregnancy. It is generally small, between 1 and 3 centimeters in diameter, although occasionally it reaches 5 centimeters or more. The fluid in the cyst is usually absorbed in the first few months of pregnancy until it disappears.

Occasionally, ovarian cysts arise from other causes. On ultrasound, it is often possible to distinguish them from a corpus luteum. They may be larger, perhaps 5 centimeters or more in diameter, and often contain septa (or partitions) inside the fluid. They may also contain solid tissue instead of fluid. Most of these are not cancerous—it is rare to have an ovarian cancer in pregnancy. Despite this, if you have a cyst that contains a solid area, you may be advised to have it removed at around 14 weeks, or earlier, if you are in severe pain.

Fibroids

Fibroids are thickenings of muscle and fibrous tissue in the wall of the uterus (see figure 4.6). They are very common, particularly in women over 40 years of age. They can become large, but they virtually never become cancerous. Large fibroids may be painful, but they do not interfere with the development or health of your fetus. Occasionally a fibroid that is low in the uterus may obstruct the birth of the baby.

Fibroids are virtually never removed in pregnancy because the muscle of the uterus has such a rich blood supply that it would be difficult to control the bleeding. The main problem with fibroids is that that they can be confused with an ovarian cyst on examination, although an ultrasound scan can diagnose them.

Other causes of pain

If you have pain during a healthy pregnancy where cysts or fibroids have been ruled out, it may come from your bowel or ligaments. These problems can rarely be detected with ultrasound. If no cause is found, it is often considered to be ligament pain, due to stretching of the ligaments that support the uterus. This pain can be a nuisance in your pregnancy, but it will ultimately settle down. It causes no disturbance to the growth or well-being of your fetus.

Common questions at 0–9 weeks of pregnancy

Where has the bleeding come from?
This is often asked when there is bleeding in early pregnancy. A scan occasionally shows a blood clot in the uterus, outside but adjacent to the pregnancy sac, where the bleeding has arisen. If there is no blood clot, the bleeding is often presumed to have come from the edge of the developing placenta.

Will the bleeding damage my unborn baby?
No. Bleeding in early pregnancy causes few, if any, long-term problems. If you do not miscarry, the fetus almost always continues to develop normally.

When did my baby die?
This question is often asked when a fetus has died in early pregnancy. The crown–rump length gives a good indication of how old your fetus was when it died. Although the cause of death is almost always unknown, couples often want to work out what they were doing at the time of death to see what could have caused it. Things like breathing paint fumes or having had several glasses of champagne may be mistakenly blamed for the death.

I know when I conceived, so why does the scan give a different date?
For convenience, a pregnancy is calculated from the first day of your last period. If you know when you conceived, tell your doctor or midwife, but by tradition and for simplicity, the pregnancy is counted from the first day of the last period. If you are certain of your dates, and a scan done in the first half of pregnancy differs from this date by more than a week, then the scan is nearly always correct.

Are my dates still correct?
Couples often ask this question after a second or subsequent scan. The earlier in pregnancy a scan is done the more accurate it is at predicting a due date. It would be inappropriate to change the date as a result of a scan done later in the pregnancy. A second scan is good at telling how the fetus is growing, but less precise at predicting a due date.

When will my baby be born?
Ultrasound can give a very accurate due date, based on the age of your fetus, but nobody can tell if the baby will be born on that day. Some babies

come very early and some very late. This unpredictable timing of the onset of labor is one of the mysteries of pregnancy.

Are my twins joined?

In a multiple pregnancy each fetus nearly always has its own separate bag of amniotic fluid surrounding it. If a membrane separating your fetuses can be seen, they are not joined.

Are my twins identical?

If twins are different sexes then they are not identical. The placenta and the membrane between the fetuses can sometimes indicate whether they are likely to be identical. They are identical if there is a very thin membrane between them early in pregnancy. If there are two placentas or the membrane is thick, then most, but not all, are non-identical. However, a single placenta is common with both identical twins and non-identical twins.

5 Prenatal testing: 10–14 weeks

New tests and scanning techniques mean it is possible to detect most of the abnormalities that can be diagnosed before birth, by the time a fetus is 13 weeks, or three months old. Many prenatal tests are now done early in pregnancy—at 10–14 weeks. The later tests of pregnancy—ultrasound, amniocentesis, and mid trimester serum screening—are still important and widely used. But there are obvious advantages of early testing. If nothing is found you can relax and enjoy your pregnancy. If an abnormality or an increased risk is found, you can make any decisions before you have announced your pregnancy to the world.

This chapter explains what to expect from the relatively new tests, such as first trimester risk assessment, now available to you (see page 56). We aim to help you understand and assess the relative advantages, disadvantages, and accuracy of these early tests.

What screening tests you are offered at this stage will often depend on your health care system and what is available locally. Some hospitals or centers routinely offer an early nuchal translucency scan or a CVS test; others do not. Some areas combine the results of your scan with your blood test; others are working towards this.

Many regions have an established 15–18 week blood screening service without a well-established nuchal translucency service; in this situation, mid trimester serum screening is likely to be your best choice. You will need advice from your doctor, or midwife about what is available locally.

What does the fetus look like at 10–14 weeks?

See Figure 5.1 for a diagram of the fetus at 12 weeks of pregnancy. It is extraordinary to see the difference on an ultrasound scan between a 10 week (see Figure 5.2) and a 12 week fetus (see Figure 5.3). The fetus grows from

3 cm (crown to rump) at 10 weeks to 5.5 cm at 12 weeks. At 10 weeks the head, body, arms and legs, fingers and toes can be seen, but details of the internal organs are not clear. By 12 weeks, most of the internal structures are visible (see figure 5.3). Because the fetus is so small, the detail depends on the quality of the pictures; this relies on how accessible the

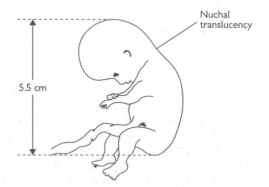

Figure 5.1 Diagram of 12 week fetus

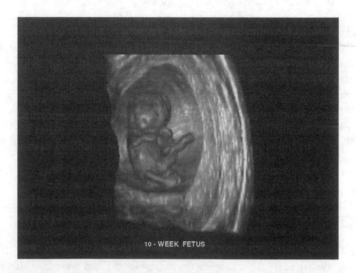

Figure 5.2 A 3D image of a 10 week fetus demonstrating that the basic fetal structure of head, body, and limbs is now developed

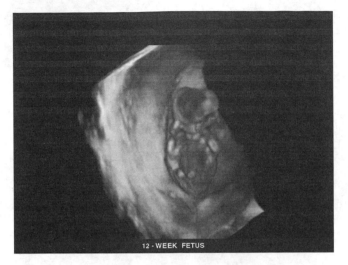

12 - WEEK FETUS

Figure 5.3 By 12 weeks improved fetal anatomy is demonstrable. Not only the external structures but most of the internal anatomy can now be identified

fetus is and the quality of the ultrasound machine. The best pictures are usually obtained with a vaginal scanner or transducer (the part of the scanner which emits the ultrasonic waves).

What tests can be done at 10–14 weeks?

At this stage of pregnancy, you have the choice of screening or diagnostic tests. A screening test such as an ultrasound scan or a blood test will give you an estimate of your risk of Down syndrome. Nuchal translucency screening was introduced in the mid to late 1990s; it is sometimes available together with early serum screening to give you a more accurate risk figure (see page 59).

An ultrasound scan at 12–13 weeks is not only a screening test for Down syndrome but can provide much more information.

A diagnostic test provides certainty that there is no chromosome abnormality. Chorionic villus sampling (CVS) is a diagnostic test that has been available since the 1980s. It can be done after 10 weeks of pregnancy and gives a definitive diagnosis of a chromosome abnormality such as Down syndrome, earlier than an amniocentesis. An early amniocentesis is possible at 12–14 weeks but is not advocated because of the higher risks at this time.

What is ultrasound?

Ultrasound is sound at a frequency so high that it cannot be heard by the human ear. Ultrasound scans involve these very high frequency sound waves being passed into the body. The reflected echoes are then analyzed to build up a picture of the internal organs, or for pregnant women, the fetus inside the uterus. It is painless and considered safe. See Chapter 7 for more on ultrasound and safety aspects.

Ultrasound is the lynch pin of prenatal testing at 10–14 weeks and later in pregnancy. Tests such as nuchal translucency scanning depend solely on ultrasound, others include ultrasound, such as the combined test of ultrasound and serum screening, whereas chorionic villus sampling requires ultrasound to guide the needle.

Screening tests such as nuchal translucency scanning and blood tests, are good but not perfect tests for the chromosome abnormalities that are commoner with increasing age, but do not screen for all chromosome abnormalities.

Risk assessment at 10–14 weeks

What is nuchal translucency scanning?

This test has quickly become a very important early ultrasound test. It was soon discovered that more accurate results were obtained from combining the nuchal translucency scan with an early blood test (see page 59 for details). Whether you are offered this depends on what is available in the area you live in.

Background

Researchers noticed that fetuses with Down syndrome detected by CVS had an increased amount of fluid under the skin behind their neck, called the nuchal fold (see Figures 5.4 a, b). The Fetal Medicine Foundation in London produced computer software that enabled the estimation of the risk of Down syndrome based on nuchal translucency measurement. Software was needed because of the other variables involved: Down syndrome increases with the age of the pregnant woman, and there are

(a)

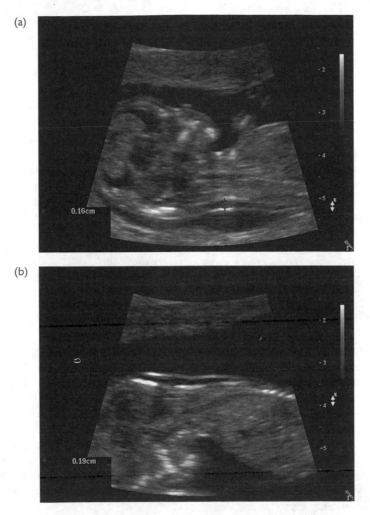

(b)

Figure 5.4 The nuchal translucency is a fluid layer beneath the skin at the back of the fetal neck. Images such as these are is used to obtain the measurement

natural increases in the thickness of the nuchal fold from 11–14 weeks. The Fetal Medicine Foundation developed a training and certification process that was offered to ultrasound providers around the world free of charge. This work by the Fetal Medicine Foundation established standards in nuchal translucency scanning. To use the software, operators must have undergone a training program and an annual audit. Trained operators are fundamental to all accurate ultrasound examinations and this procedure is now being used worldwide. Some groups have produced their own software.

How is the test done?

For this test, the fetus must have a crown–rump length (CRL) of between 4.5–8.2 cm. That is, it must be over 11 weeks but a maximum of 14 weeks old. To get an accurate nuchal translucency measurement you need excellent ultrasound equipment.

For nine out of 10 women the measurement of the nuchal translucency is best done by a scan through your abdomen. The measurement must be taken with the fetus either facing straight up to the scanner or facing directly away. The operator will need to move their hand around your abdomen to obtain this precise angle.

A vaginal scan is used for about one in 10 women, when a nuchal translucency measurement cannot be obtained through the abdomen. Vaginal scanning is not usually the best way of taking this measurement as the fetus is approached from one direction only.

How accurate is the nuchal translucency scan in detecting Down syndrome?

Like all screening tests, nuchal translucency scans are not perfect. Initial results suggested that approximately eight out of 10 fetuses with Down syndrome are detected by this type of scan. More recent studies have suggested a lower detection rate for Down syndrome using nuchal translucency. Some suggested a figure as low as six out of 10.

If your risk of having a Down syndrome baby is found to be one in 300 or higher, such as one in 200 or one in 100, you are told you are at increased risk. If your risk is found to be lower, such as one in 400 or one in 500, you are told you are low risk. Approximately 8 per cent or one in 12 women are told they are in the increased risk group for Down syndrome after a nuchal translucency scan.

Most of these women go on to have healthy normal babies; and the test result is called 'false positive'. Being told you are at increased risk puts great stress on pregnant women and makes any decision about further tests even more agonising. Screening tests for Down syndrome can also have 'false negative' results—some women who are told they are at low risk do go on to have a Down syndrome baby.

This detection rate for Down syndrome can be improved by having an early blood test, called serum screening, as well as the nuchal translucency scan (see combined screening, below). A major advantage of combining a nuchal translucency scan with a blood test is that fewer women are found to be in the at risk group—around 5 per cent or one in 20. This is the same number that are found at mid trimester serum screening (see chapter 6).

Refinements to these tests are ongoing. Computer software is being developed that allows the nasal bone to be included in testing. Down syndrome fetuses often have a delay in developing nasal bone; if none is seen the chance of Down syndrome being present is increased.

Early (first trimester) serum screening

Researchers set out to investigate whether a serum, or blood test, similar to the 15–18 week test, could be used to screen much earlier pregnancies for Down syndrome. They looked at a large range of different substances present in the blood in the first three months of pregnancy and found two that might be suitable for Down syndrome screening early in pregnancy—free beta-hCG and PAPP-A. For best results, blood should be taken at 10–11 weeks. This is because one of the substances, PAPP-A, performs better at that time. While these blood tests were not accurate enough to use alone, a much better test was developed by taking these results and adding them to the nuchal translucency results.

Combined nuchal translucency and early blood test

Your risk of having a Down syndrome baby can be more accurately assessed if you have an early blood test combined with a nuchal translucency test. Taking the early blood test results and adding these into the nuchal translucency software results in nine out of 10 Down syndrome fetuses being detected.

Combining a scan and a blood test is more accurate at identifying abnormalities, but it does add some organisational difficulties. The blood is often taken at 10–11 weeks, and the ultrasound at 12–13 weeks. The blood test results are not given alone as the risk figures are combined.

Some hospitals or centres have developed a 'one-stop shop'. This simplifies the organization, and allows women to have the blood test and scan together and to get the results all on the same day. This relies on having a high quality pathology laboratory very close to the ultrasound center.

Integrated screening test

At some hospitals or centers you may be offered integrated screening, where the results of different tests are combined. You may have a nuchal translucency scan at 12 weeks, and instead of getting your result then, you wait until after your blood test at 15–18 weeks. The two results are combined to give your risk figure. As the later blood test has better results than the early one, this is a very effective test, detecting around 94 per cent of Down syndrome fetuses. Another type of integrated screening might involve the nuchal translucency scan, plus the early and late blood tests. Integrated tests may not be widely available in all areas.

Waiting almost a month for your test results and your risk figure can be difficult for many women. You will have seen the ultrasound images from your nuchal translucency scan, yet you are denied knowledge of the result. This runs counter to the philosophy of prenatal testing that advocates open and free communication with the pregnant woman at all times. But it has the advantage of a slightly higher detection rate for Down syndrome.

A different and more problematic sort of integrated test is having early screening for Down syndrome by whatever means, and then looking for 'markers' on ultrasound at 18–22 weeks. 'Markers' are any changes in a fetus that might or might not indicate an abnormality. If a marker is found that might increase your risk of Down syndrome, this can be added to your previous calculation to give you a new risk figure.

Problems arise if pregnant women are just told about the new marker, and not given a new risk figure. It can be frightening to be told that a marker has been found at your 18–22 week scan, especially if a previous screening test showed you were at low risk. The resulting anxiety is often unnecessary, as an unexpected case of Down syndrome is rarely identified this way.

If the presence of a marker is used to recalculate your risk of Down syndrome, it can be difficult deciding what multiplication factor to use; different figures are available. See Chapter 7, page 119 for more on markers.

Integrated screening is only acceptable if the various risks are multiplied to give you a single final risk.

What else is early ultrasound used for?

Detecting trisomies

Women in their late 30s and 40s often think they have a higher chance of having a baby with all sorts of abnormalities. In fact, their chance of most abnormalities is not increased. But they are at increased risk of chromosomal abnormalities called autosomal trisomies.

Our chromosomes are in pairs with 23 pairs making a total of 46 chromosomes in every cell. If there is an extra chromosome to make a total of 47, then the extra chromosome is usually either chromosome 21 (Down syndrome, the commonest chromosome abnormality), chromosome 18 (trisomy 18 or Edward syndrome) or chromosome 13 (trisomy 13 or Patau syndrome). Fetuses with any of these three chromosome abnormalities tend to have a thickened nuchal translucency and are commonly detected with the nuchal translucency scan or the combined test. The nuchal translucency software gives a risk for trisomy 18 or 13 and the combined test also includes a risk figure for trisomy 18. Trisomy 18 and 13 produce far more devastating effects than Down syndrome. Affected fetuses usually have a wide range of physical abnormalities and most will die during pregnancy or immediately after birth.

Collectively, trisomy 21, 18, and 13 cause about 70 per cent of the chromosome abnormalities detected before birth. The remaining 30 per cent are often, but not always, less severe and they are not age related. They are as common in 20 year olds as in 40 year olds. Most of this remaining 30 per cent are not detected on either ultrasound or any blood tests. They can only be identified prenatally by amniocentesis or CVS.

Dating the pregnancy

In the first 3 months of pregnancy, fetuses grow very quickly and at a similar rate—it is unusual to find significant differences in size between different fetuses at this early stage. Early scans are therefore the best time to date a pregnancy, certainly better than relying on menstrual dates and even better than a later scan.

Diagnosing multiple pregnancy

It is a great advantage to diagnose multiple pregnancies early so that chorionicity can be determined (see Chapter 4, page 46).

Diagnosing pregnancy failure or miscarriage

Sadly, at a 12 week scan, one in 50 women find that their fetus has died. Often, there are no outward signs and neither you nor your doctor or midwife will have had any suspicions or worries. The fetus may have died some time ago without you having any bleeding.

Many women think that miscarriage involves heavy bleeding and because of the bleeding the pregnancy comes away, causing the death of the fetus. Women often wonder why the dead fetus stayed inside and was not miscarried naturally. In fact, miscarriage usually occurs because the fetal heart stops beating. After about a week some of the pregnancy symptoms improve, particularly if there has been nausea and vomiting. This can be confusing because the vomiting often improves at around 2–3 months anyway. The symptoms improve because hormone production from the placenta starts to drop after the fetus has died. Eventually, some weeks or months later, the hormone levels drop sufficiently for bleeding to start, and this ends in miscarriage.

Since many scans are now being performed at 12–13 weeks, it is possible that your scan occurs in the time after your fetus has died, but before bleeding has started.

Detecting physical abnormalities

The best time to scan for physical abnormalities is 18–22 weeks (see Chapter 7). Although magnificent images can be obtained of the anatomy of a tiny 12–13 week old fetus, more physical abnormalities can be seen when it is bigger. Even if the structures appear normal at this early stage, pregnant women will be offered another scan at 18–22 weeks as two or three in 10 physical abnormalities can be missed at this stage.

Despite this, 70–80 per cent of the abnormalities that would be found at 18–20 weeks can be picked up by scanning at 12–13 weeks A high detection rate of abnormalities at this early stage depends on:

1) A high quality ultrasound scanner. If there are technical difficulties with the scan—and there often are—good equipment enhances the ability to detect abnormalities early.

2) An experienced operator.

The limits of ultrasound in detecting physical abnormalities at 10–14 weeks

A scan at 10–14 weeks cannot detect all physical abnormalities because:

The fetal structures are very small early on, so abnormalities are harder to pick up. Despite this, even most of the major heart abnormalities, commonly the most difficult abnormalities to diagnose, can be picked at 12–13 weeks.

Some abnormalities, or signs of abnormalities, evolve after 13 weeks. Some examples include water on the brain (hydrocephaly) and a blockage to urine flow from the kidneys (hydronephrosis). Abnormalities where there is reduced growth usually only develop after 13 weeks—for example short limbs (dwarfism), or a small head (microcephaly).

Although an abnormality might be present at 12 weeks, the signs that are used to diagnose the abnormality may not be present. This applies particularly for spina bifida where seeing the spina bifida itself can be very difficult early on. But by 18 weeks there are relatively easily detectable changes in the brain and skull shape that are used as indicators that spina bifida is likely to be present. These head signs are not present at 13 weeks.

3) A vaginal scan—if the fetus is accessible to a vaginal scanner, views will always be better than with an abdominal scanner. Sometimes the uterus is sitting high up in the abdomen and the fetus is too far away from the vaginal scanner, so an abdominal scanner has to be used.

4) Good luck—good views depend on the fetus happening to lie in an accessible position with plenty of fluid around it, preferably facing towards the scanner.

5) Gestational age—it is difficult or impossible to obtain good quality views at 10–11 weeks. Far better detail is seen at 12–13 weeks and more abnormalities can be picked at this time.

Seeing the physical structure of your fetus at 12–13 weeks can give you wonderful reassurance that all is normal, but some abnormalities that can be picked at 18–20 weeks will be missed at an early scan.

What is chorionic villus sampling (CVS)?

Chorionic (pronounced ko-re-on-ik) villus sampling involves passing a needle or tube into the placenta and withdrawing a few small fragments of the tissue into a syringe. It is called 'chorionic' because the chorion is the name for the placenta in the very early stages of pregnancy. The name 'villus' comes from the microscopic appearance of the chorionic surface—large numbers of finger-like structures or 'villi' project outwards towards the lining of the uterus. Chorionic villus sampling is occasionally called 'placental biopsy'.

CVS and amniocentesis are the two commonly used tests that allow Down syndrome and other chromosomal abnormalities to be diagnosed with certainty. They also aid the diagnosis of some genetic diseases for many at risk couples. Many hospitals and centers have found a swing away from amniocentesis to CVS. The attraction of CVS is that the results are available very much earlier in pregnancy. It is often suggested that there is a greater risk of miscarriage with CVS, in fact, if it is done by an experienced doctor, there is little if any difference in the risk.

CVS was first used in Denmark in 1968, but was abandoned because it caused too many miscarriages. It was used in China to determine the sex of a fetus early in pregnancy. It was first used to test for abnormalities in the USSR in 1982 and afterwards in Europe. Initially, all specimens were taken by passing a smooth tube through the vagina and the cervix and up into the uterus. But in 1984, successful attempts were made to pass a needle through the abdominal wall and uterus and then into the placenta.

When CVS was first used, different methods of obtaining placental tissue were tried with different success rates. Some high rates of miscarriage were reported. Techniques have now been refined and only those methods with a low miscarriage rate are used. If CVS is performed by an experienced doctor, it is now believed to increase your chance of miscarriage by a maximum of 1 per cent.

Why have CVS?

CVS and amniocentesis are usually offered to pregnant women who are at increased risk of having a baby with specific abnormalities. They are not general tests to see if your fetus is normal. If you want to check the fetal chromosomes there is a choice of CVS or amniocentesis, as they test for the same conditions. The only difference is that amniocentesis can also test for spina bifida. But, as ultrasound is now the main method of diagnosing spina bifida, this is rarely important.

While there are a host of genetic diseases that can be tested by analyzing chorionic villi, most of the diseases are rare. They will be looked for only if there is a family history, or if testing has shown that a couple are at risk of a disorder which could be passed on to their children.

You might want to consider CVS to check your chromosomes if you fall into any of the following at risk groups:

1. You are in your late thirties or forties—so are at greater risk of having a Down syndrome baby.
2. Your nuchal translucency scan or your early serum screening showed you are at increased risk of chromosome abnormality.
3. You have previously had a baby with a chromosomal abnormality.

Sometimes low risk women women simply want to be certain that the fetal chromosomes are normal. In some medical systems it can be difficult for low risk women to get CVS or an amniocentesis.

Joan was sent to a specialist clinic to discuss prenatal diagnosis. She was 34 years old and felt disconcerted at having been sent along as she 'didn't think she was old enough' to need to consider invasive testing with CVS or amniocentesis. Joan's prime concern was whether it was appropriate for her doctor to have raised the issue of testing. Initial discussion focused on who should be offered prenatal diagnosis. Joan was aware that in her region women are routinely offered prenatal diagnosis if they are 37 years or more at the time of the delivery. She was unaware that that elsewhere, 35 was a more common minimum age. Discussion soon turned to whether some government committee should dictate who is eligible for prenatal diagnosis, whether the doctor should decide, or whether prenatal diagnosis should be available to all pregnant women who understand the risks.

When is the best time for CVS?

CVS can be performed any time from 10 weeks. By 10 weeks the placenta thickens in one area, and it is possible to identify where the fully formed placenta will be situated.

If you are 15 weeks pregnant or more, amniocentesis is usually considered your best option, although some hospitals and centers still perform CVS, believing that there is no difference in the risk of these tests.

An initial test result—sometimes called FISH by medical staff (see page 74)—can be available within 2 days. The laboratory needs up to 2 weeks to fully process your specimen. Your results should be available at 12 weeks of pregnancy or soon after. At this time you do not look pregnant and have not felt movements. If you are unfortunate enough to have an abnormality detected and you have an abortion, it is still early enough to dilate the cervix and carry out a simple suction curettage procedure. It takes only a few minutes and an overnight stay in hospital is usually unnecessary.

Who will perform the CVS and what are the risks?

Before making your decision on amniocentesis or on transabdominal or transcervical CVS (see page 66), you should ask your obstetrician, doctor or midwife about the techniques that local experts perform regularly. A United States study found that doctors need to perform approximately 75 CVS tests in order to learn the technique. Their performance improves considerably with experience. Independent follow-up of women who have undergone CVS has shown miscarriage rates as high as 20 per cent. These high rates are often due to the inexperience of the operators, and highlight the importance of selecting the best expertise available. It has been suggested that skill improves after the first 100 cases of transabdominal CVS, and after the first 300 transcervical tests. To maintain their expertise, a doctor performing CVS should do at least 50 procedures per year.

You can ask the doctor performing the CVS how many patients miscarry after the procedure in his or her experience. Experienced centers often quote 1 per cent as the maximum miscarriage rate for CVS. On top of this, there is the 'background' risk—even without the test about 2.5 per cent of women whose pregnancy appears normal at 10 weeks will miscarry. This background risk increases with the age of the pregnant woman.

What happens before a CVS?

If there is any doubt about the age of your pregnancy or if you have had a complication such as bleeding, you might be offered an ultrasound scan some time before your CVS.

No special preparation is needed on the day of the CVS. You may be asked to have some urine in your bladder either for the ultrasound or for the CVS, particularly for transcervical CVS.

The ultrasound is carried out in the usual way, followed immediately by the CVS, without you having to move from the examination couch. The doctor will want to know your blood group. This is because some blood cells from the fetus may cross into your own circulation during the procedure. If you are one of the 15 per cent of women who are Rh-negative, your body might produce antibodies to these cells, which can cause problems in subsequent pregnancies. Women with a Rh-negative blood group will be given an 'anti-D' (or Rhogam) injection to prevent this happening.

How is the CVS test done?

There are two ways of passing a needle into the developing placenta:

1. A blunt tube (called a cannula) or fine forceps is passed through the cervix and into the uterus to the developing placenta; this is called a transcervical CVS (see Figure 5.5).

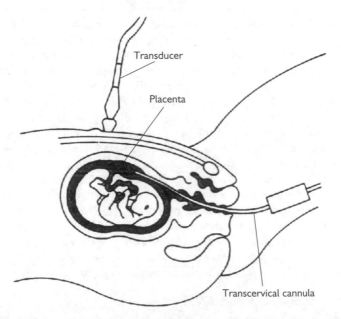

Figure 5.5 Chorionic villus sampling (CVS), using the transcervical method: a cannula is passed up through the cervix then guided into the placenta with ultrasound

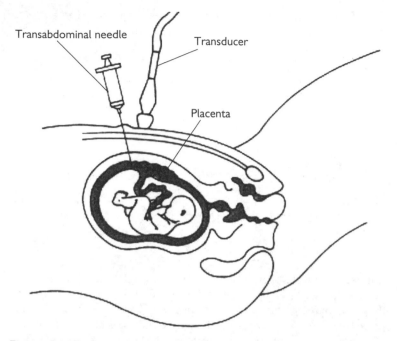

Transabdominal needle

Transducer

Placenta

Figure 5.6 Chorionic villus sampling (CVS), using the transabdominal method: a needle is passed through the abdomen down into the placenta

2. A fine needle is passed through the skin of the abdominal wall, through the uterus and down into the placenta. This is called a transabdominal CVS (see Figure 5.6). From the pregnant woman's point of view, this is very similar to an amniocentesis.

Which method is used depends partly on medical factors (see Table 5.1 below) but above all, on the expertise of the operator.

What happens during a transcervical CVS?

For a transcervical CVS your bladder must be full. Before the test you will have a scan and your doctor will check that there is enough urine in your bladder. You will then be asked to lie on your back, with your legs lifted and apart, at the foot of the examining table. After washing in and around the vagina with an antiseptic solution the doctor passes a speculum—a metal or plastic object which holds the walls of the vagina apart—into the vagina to view the cervix. Having located the cervix, the doctor may grasp

Table 5.1 Factors influencing the choice between transabdominal and transcervical CVS

	Transcervical	Transabdominal
Access:		
—cervical fibroid	Difficult	No difficulty
—sharply retroverted uterus	May be difficult	May be difficult
—sharply anteverted uterus	May be difficult	No difficulty
Vaginal infection	Avoid	No problem
Risk of test*	Low in experienced hands	Low in experienced hands

* The most important determinant of risk is the experience and expertise of the doctor performing the test

it if necessary with a pair of forceps. You may feel a pinching sensation. The specimen is taken by passing a blunt tube or fine forceps up through the cervix into the uterus, and advancing it into the developing placental tissue (see Figure 5.5). By placing the ultrasound transducer onto the skin of your abdomen, the doctor is able to watch the tube or forceps passing through the cervix, and carefully guide it into the placenta. An anaesthetic is not used. Any irregularity of the wall of the uterus can usually be negotiated by careful and gentle manipulation.

Most women feel very little as the tube or forceps is passed into the uterus because even in pregnancy, the cervix is sufficiently open to allow its passage. If a tube or cannula is used, suction is applied to a syringe at the other end and the tip is moved around within the placenta to obtain some tissue. The cannula is then withdrawn, the tissue ejected from the syringe and inspected to see if there is enough. If there are not enough villi in the specimen, the test can be repeated by passing a second cannula through the cervix. If fine forceps are used, the technique is essentially the same, except that a small piece of placental tissue is grasped with the teeth of the forceps.

How often it is necessary to repeat the test depends on the experience of the operator. If there is not enough material after two or three attempts, the procedure will usually be rescheduled. Continuing to repeat the test on the same day increases the risk of miscarriage. The pregnancy and the fetal heartbeat are rechecked after the test. Once the CVS has been completed, you may remain on the examining table for a short time before emptying your bladder. There may be some slight vaginal bleeding. You may be advised to sit and relax for a while before going home.

What happens during a transabdominal CVS?

You do not need a full bladder for the transabdominal CVS. First, you lie on your back on the examining table while an ultrasound examination is carried out. You remain lying down for the CVS. Using ultrasound, the doctor locates the best place to pass the needle through your skin and, if a local anaesthetic is to be used, it is injected into that site. Local anaesthetic can be injected into the surface of the skin and the layers immediately beneath. It is more difficult to anaesthetize the layers deep inside the abdomen, and discomfort from the test is usually from these deeper layers.

The specimen is taken by passing a needle down through the wall of your abdomen as shown in Figure 5.6, and into the placenta. The needle is carefully guided by watching it with ultrasound. Some operators use an attachment at the side of the ultrasound transducer to hold the needle on a predetermined course—and the course is shown on the screen as a dotted line. An alternative technique is to hold the transducer at a distance from the needle to watch its advance. The best method is the one which the operator is most comfortable with.

Once the needle tip is through the wall of the uterus and inside the placental tissue, a sample can be taken. This can be done by applying suction to a syringe at the other end of the needle, or by feeding a second needle inside the first while applying suction with a syringe at the other end. With the two-needle method, repeated amounts are taken from the fine needle until enough material is obtained. After the test, the pregnancy and the fetal heartbeat are checked before you leave the room.

The laboratory likes to receive at least 10 mg of tissue for analysis. This amount of tissue is visible to the naked eye and looks like a few flecks floating in the fluid at the bottom of a flask. It should be taken the same day to the laboratory for processing.

Which method of CVS is best?

Minor variations to the techniques described are used at different hospitals or centers. A wide variety of needles are used. There are advantages and disadvantages of each technique; it ultimately comes down to the personal preference of the doctor. Even if you would prefer a particular approach, it is usually better to have whatever method is offered. If a doctor is asked to change his or her technique, the results may not be as good. You would do better to change to a doctor who uses the method you prefer rather than asking your own doctor to change their method.

Does a CVS test hurt?

Whatever method of CVS is used, is not a painful test for most women. In the transcervical test, some women find having a full bladder uncomfortable, and the vaginal examination disturbing. If an instrument is used to grasp the cervix, it might cause discomfort. Usually the passage of the cannula into the placenta is not particularly unpleasant.

If the CVS is transabdominal, it is usually tolerated well. It is similar to an amniocentesis, and although a slightly wider needle is used, it is not usually painful. In a survey of 50 women who had transabdominal CVS in Melbourne, Australia, 90 per cent reported no pain or only mild pain. The other 10 per cent described the pain as moderate and none reported severe pain. In rare cases there can be pain if the uterus is tilted backwards and the placenta is in the far wall of the uterus. This makes it more difficult to reach with the needle.

In the Australian study of 50 women, 17 (or 34 per cent), developed abdominal discomfort after the transabdominal CVS. This was described as mild by 13, moderate by 3, and severe by 1. The pain was described as similar to uterine contractions. It began between 1 and 15 minutes after the CVS and lasted between 2 and 20 minutes.

What will happen after the CVS test?

After the test you will be advised to wait for a short time before you go home. You will be quite capable of driving yourself home, but you might prefer to have somebody with you. Many women feel tired and emotionally drained after CVS, as they have been psychologically preparing for the test for some time. After any test in which a needle is passed into the uterus, it is a good idea to relax at home for the rest of the day, although there should be no reason to go to bed. Most doctors say you can continue with your normal activities the following day and for the rest of your pregnancy.

After a transcervical CVS you can have bleeding from the vagina which is coming from the cervix or the uterus itself. This bleeding is usually over very quickly, but may be followed by some brown staining for a day or two as the last of the blood drains away.

Bleeding is rare after transabdominal CVS as the lower part of the uterus has not been disturbed. Some women have discomfort in their lower abdomen for a short time after the test. This nearly always settles quickly and is not linked to any risk of miscarriage or damage to the developing pregnancy.

It is rare to have any other problems after a CVS test. If you do have any other symptoms, such as continued bleeding, pain or loss of fluid, it is important that you contact your doctor. Even if you are unlucky enough to have any of these symptoms, they are likely to settle and your pregnancy should continue unaffected.

Two women who have undergone CVS give their impressions of the procedure:

I had another surprise pregnancy and this time I chose a CVS. It would only involve a curette rather than going through labor if a termination was necessary. From my reading, the risks weren't that much greater than amniocentesis. The procedure amazed me. The needle went through my abdomen, into the uterus and was dipped in and out. This had to be done four or five times, but it was not painful. I was quite philosophical about it. The pregnancy was unexpected and if it wasn't to be, then I would cope with that when the time came.

When I found out I was pregnant, I went to the gynaecologist quickly because I wanted to have a CVS. I had heard it was the same procedure as amniocentesis but that it was done earlier at 10 weeks. I found the risk of miscarriage of 1 per cent quite acceptable. Initially, my husband was against the test because he didn't want me to terminate the pregnancy if the baby was found to have Down syndrome. When I explained how a disabled child would reduce the amount of attention we could show our daughter, he mellowed. The actual test was frightening but straightforward. The needle only had to go in once and there was no pain, just discomfort. It was wonderful having test results back so early because it relieved all the pressures.

What are the risks of CVS?

The thought of passing a needle into the placenta with its very rich blood supply is frightening. Anybody who has seen the large blood vessels leading to the placenta would expect such a test to cause severe bleeding. Clinical trials have shown that this rarely happens with CVS.

Complications of any procedure may be immediate or occur some time later. Immediate complications with CVS may be pain or failure to obtain a specimen. Some slight bleeding is common after transcervical CVS, but is rare after transabdominal CVS. The bleeding usually settles within a few days. The most important delayed complication of CVS is miscarriage (see following page).

There is very little chance of directly hurting the fetus as the needle does not enter the amniotic sac. It is possible to rupture the pregnancy sac at the time of the test, but this is rare with an experienced operator. If this happens during a transcervical CVS you may miscarry because the cannula leaves such a large hole. It is less likely to cause any complications if it happens during a transabdominal CVS as the needle is much finer. Another rare complication is the formation of a clot at the place where the specimen was taken from. If this happens it will usually resolve without causing any problem.

Significant complications other than miscarriages are rare following CVS. There is no damage to the placenta in the short or the long term. If the placenta is examined after CVS it is difficult to find any sign of the test. Your fetus will grow just as well after CVS as those that have not had the test.

Miscarriage

The main risk of CVS is miscarriage. It is difficult to know the exact risk of CVS causing a miscarriage. If a fetus is alive at 10 weeks there is a 2.5 per cent chance that it will miscarry anyway without being tested. The chance of miscarriage unrelated to CVS increases with the age of the pregnant woman. If she is 37 years or more, the figure rises (see Chapter 4, page 45 on miscarriage).

If CVS is performed by an experienced doctor, who has done many of these tests, the miscarriage risk is estimated at a maximum of 1 per cent. To find out the true risk of miscarriage due to CVS, a study would need to be done in which women were randomly given either CVS or no testing at all and the miscarriage rates compared. This type of study is impossible as couples have the right to choose to have a test or not.

Two studies, one from Canada and one from the USA, compared the miscarriage rate after transcervical CVS to that after amniocentesis. One found that CVS caused 0.6 per cent and the other 0.8 per cent more miscarriages than amniocentesis. Some units produced better and some worse results than this—emphasizing the point that the risk depends on who performs the test. A subsequent USA study of many of the same operators showed that with continued experience, the risks came close to those of amniocentesis. A Danish study showed transabdominal CVS had a similar risk of miscarriage to amniocentesis, but a higher risk with transcervical CVS. The most important factor with both is the experience of the operator.

If you do miscarry after the test, there is usually no way of telling whether the test was responsible as the symptoms are identical to those of any other miscarriage. The first thing you will notice is bleeding. Your doctor may then suggest you have an ultrasound scan to check whether your fetus is still alive. If it is alive then you should rest until the bleeding stops. If you do miscarry it is not possible to predict when it will happen. Sadly, a miscarriage can occur at any time during your pregnancy, whether you have a test or not. It is more common earlier in a pregnancy, so if you have a miscarriage around the time of a CVS test it is impossible to know if it would have happened anyway.

A slightly higher risk of miscarriage is usually quoted for CVS than amniocentesis. Common figures quoted are up to 1 per cent for CVS and up to half a per cent for amniocentesis. These risks are very operator-dependent. Experienced operators performing large numbers of tests can achieve a miscarriage rate following CVS at least as low as amniocentesis.

Other complications

One rare complication is severe infection following transcervical CVS, resulting in miscarriage and severe illness in the pregnant woman. Because of this, transcervical CVS will not be done if you have an untreated infection in your cervix. This is very rare—no cases occurred in the 2235 women who underwent transcervical CVS in the USA study quoted above.

It has been suggested that 'amputation' type defects of the arms and legs can follow CVS. These reports included babies born with missing fingers, toes, or lower parts of the arm or leg, and it caused a major scare. These limb abnormalities were reported by inexperienced operators, who were performing CVS before 9 weeks of pregnancy.

The conclusion of a group of experts, including the World Health Organization, was that 'present evidence of an increased incidence of limb reduction defects is consistent with an association of very early sampling (at or before 8 menstrual weeks) with some fetal limb abnormalities. There is no evidence to suggest an increased risk of congenital malformation when the CVS is performed after the 8th completed menstrual week.'

Today, CVS is not usually performed before 10 weeks, and it should always be done by an experienced operator. When CVS is done under these conditions there is no known increased risk of limb abnormalities.

What happens to the sample and when do I get my results?

When the placental tissue that has been collected—the aim is at least 10 mg—is taken to the laboratory, the placental villi are carefully dissected to remove any decidual cells, that is, cells from the lining of the pregnant woman's uterus.

Either or both of the following methods are then used for analysis:

1. The chromosomes are looked at either without culturing or by culturing for a short period of up to 24 hours. This method analyzes the

lining cells of the villi of the placenta—called the cytotrophoblastic cells. You get a result very quickly, usually within 2 days.

2. The specimen is cultured for 1 week or more before processing. The cells are taken from the incubator and analyzed when enough cell colonies have grown. This method analyzes the core of the villi—called the mesenchymal cells. It is the most detailed and most accurate assessment for chromosome abnormality. You wait 7 to 14 days for a result.

In the early days of CVS the first method was used. However, it was discovered that occasionally the chromosome result was different to that of the fetus. Many laboratories now use the rapid method, and follow up with the long-term method to confirm the results. Others use only the long-term method. For complex reasons associated with the early development of these two tissues, the chromosomes can occasionally differ.

The time taken to process the results varies with the technique used by the laboratory. Work on the samples is time-consuming, with one technician processing only about five a week. Overload on laboratory resources often delays the results. Generally, the result is available by 13 weeks of pregnancy—much earlier than amniocentesis.

Testing with FISH or PCR

FISH (fluorescence in situ hybridization) and PCR (polymerase chain reaction) are DNA tests. These techniques allow a very quick way to test for the most common chromosome abnormalities because they can be performed directly on the specimen without the need for lengthy cell culture. Results are usually available within 24 to 48 hours.

FISH works by using a coloured fluorescent label that attaches to a specific piece of chromosomal DNA within the cell. Cells from a person with normal chromosomes will show two fluorescent spots within each cell that represent the pair of chromosomes being tested. An individual with Down syndrome will show three fluorescent spots because there are three copies of chromosome 21 instead of the usual two. The most common FISH test uses five different labels and can exclude about 90 per cent of significant chromosome abnormalities by testing for chromosome 21, as well as trisomy 13 and 18 and the loss or gain of the sex chromosomes (chromosomes X and Y). Because of the cost involved, FISH is only used to test for these major abnormalities unless there is a special reason to test for something else.

PCR is an alternative method of rapidly testing for common chromosome abnormalities in amniocentesis and CVS specimens. The PCR test works by isolating and then multiplying very small amounts of DNA that has been extracted from the cells. This amplified DNA is then tested on a special machine that checks the number of chromosomes present. Both FISH and PCR are very efficient at quickly screening for the common chromosome abnormalities and the choice of test usually rests with the preference and expertise of the testing laboratory. PCR is more amenable to large scale testing and is therefore more common in larger, centralised laboratories.

It is important to realize that FISH and PCR only test for a specific group of chromosome abnormalities—the most common ones. The traditional culture method described at 2. on the page opposite, is always done as well as FISH, since this allows every chromosome to be fully analysed.

DNA testing is also available to couples whose pregnancy is at risk of a specific gene defect. These include cystic fibrosis and fragile X syndrome. Many other diseases can be tested for, and this number increases each year. Each disease tested is expensive so these tests are not usually offered unless there is a specific reason to do so. The most common reason is that the couple or a close relative already has a child affected by the disease.

Does CVS always produce a result?

There are two main reasons why CVS can fail to produce a result. Either the operator failed to obtain an adequate specimen—called technical failure, or the laboratory failed to produce an adequate result—called laboratory failure.

Both of these failure rates are higher with CVS than with amniocentesis, as CVS can be a more difficult technique. Less than 1 per cent of women who have an amniocentesis will need a repeat test, whereas 2 per cent of women who have had CVS carried out by an expert, will need a repeat test.

With experience, the operator learns ways round the difficulties or can anticipate problems that could result in a failed test. Even so, experienced operators have a failure rate of between 1 per cent and 6 per cent for transcervical CVS and about 1.5 per cent for transabdominal CVS.

Occasionally the laboratory receives a good specimen but none of the cells from the placenta grow. This happens in 1–2 specimens in 1000 and prevents chromosome analysis. If the growth does fail, the alternatives are to repeat the CVS or have an amniocentesis. Whichever of the two methods is chosen, it is unlikely that the second specimen would fail to grow.

Confusing results

There are two other potential sources of error which can cause confusing results. Maternal cell contamination is when cells from the pregnant woman grow, rather than cells from the fetus. This rarely happens, because laboratories have become experienced at processing samples and meticulously removing any of the pregnant woman's tissues from the specimen. Another occasional problem is mosaicism, when different cells analyzed in the laboratory have different chromosomes. This condition affects a small percentage of people. The outcome for the baby depends on what the chromosome types are and the proportion of each type of cell. The CVS may occasionally show mosaicism that is not present in the fetus. This is called confined placental mosaicism because it is confined to the placenta; it is not in the fetus. Experts often have a good idea whether mosaicism is likely to be affecting the fetus by looking at the pattern of the mixture of cells. Some mixtures of cells that are seen after CVS are so rare in liveborn babies that further testing usually shows that it is not present. Mosaicism occurs in approximately 1 per cent of CVS tests and can readily be sorted out if an amniocentesis is performed.

Occasionally the test results are ambiguous or later prove to be incorrect. These may be 'false positive', when an abnormal result is obtained for a normal fetus, or 'false negative', when a normal result is obtained in a fetus with abnormal chromosomes. Most false positive results are quickly detected by the laboratory, as the chromosome abnormality is not seen in live fetuses, and a follow-up amniocentesis is recommended. False negatives are very rare with CVS.

Table 5.2 below gives the figures for the different CVS failures. It shows that 2 per cent of women will require further testing either with a repeat CVS or amniocentesis. Whether or not further testing is required depends mostly on the expertise of the doctor, as failure to obtain a suitable specimin is potentially the largest group. Failure rates are at the lower end of the range in most experienced centers. It is important to discuss these matters with your doctor to find out what the experience is in your region.

CVS in multiple pregnancies

CVS can be done in twin pregnancies, but some operators are not happy to perform CVS on twins. It is not usually recommended if there are three

Table 5.2 Reasons for failure of CVS testing

Inadequate or no specimen	1–6%
Cells do not grow	0.2%
Doubtful result	0.8–2%
Total	**2%**

or more fetuses. Access to the separate placentas may be difficult—increasingly so with each extra fetus. It is reasonable to perform CVS on twins if the placenta of each fetus is accessible.

If a chromosome abnormality is found most women choose to have a fetal reduction—an injection of a salt solution into the heart of the affected fetus. Care must be taken at the time of the CVS to map out the position of the sacs so the operator can later be certain which fetus is affected (see Chapter 9 for details of termination procedures).

If you have twins and want CVS we recommend that you discuss your suitability for CVS with your doctor.

What is an early amniocentesis?

Amniocentesis is considered early when it is carried out before the traditional time of 15 weeks. Most early amnioceneses are carried out at 12–14 weeks. Skilled operators can reliably perform amniocentesis at this earlier time, although there can be more technical difficulties. The amniotic membrane that surrounds the fetus is not fully fused with the wall of the uterus. Therefore when the operator attempts to pass a needle through the amniotic membrane it can indent on the tip of the needle instead of the needle passing through it. This can usually be overcome with careful selection of the site of the amniocentesis and rapid passage of the needle.

The major problem with early amniocentesis is that the risks are higher. There is a higher chance of miscarriage and a higher chance of amniotic fluid leakage—the loss of amniotic fluid through the vagina after the test. CVS is a safer test than amniocentesis at this time. Since CVS is harder to learn, some operators prefer early amniocentesis.

Questions about chorionic villus sampling

Does CVS cause my fetus to move?
During CVS you may see your fetus moving on the ultrasound screen, but these movements are spontaneous—CVS has no influence on them. The needle is outside the pregnancy sac, so the fetus does not have any sensation or awareness of its presence.

Is CVS as accurate as amniocentesis?
If the result is 'abnormal' with either test, this result can be relied upon to be accurate. Some 'normal' CVS results can be doubtful; having an amniocentesis later can nearly always clear them up.

Can CVS detect as much as amniocentesis?
With very rare exceptions these two tests are as good as each other for diagnosing chromosomal abnormalities. Spina bifida cannot be diagnosed by
CVS, but most women who have CVS are at low risk of having a baby with
spina bifida. Ultrasound is now the prime method of diagnosing spina
bifida.

Do more people choose CVS or amniocentesis?
The most popular choice depends on local expertise. Where there is local
expertise in CVS it is found that more and more women are choosing this
method because of the early results.

Can I have CVS if I have been bleeding?
If you have vaginal bleeding in early pregnancy you have an increased
chance of miscarriage, even when your pregnancy appears healthy on
ultrasound. Your 'background' risk is higher than if you had no bleeding.
It is uncertain whether performing a CVS in this situation results in an
increased risk of miscarriage. If you have had no bleeding in the week
before the proposed CVS, and your pregnancy appears healthy on ultrasound, then the test is unlikely to cause an increased risk of miscarriage.

If CVS causes a miscarriage when would it happen?
There is no clear answer to this question. A miscarriage can happen at any
time and there is no way of telling if the CVS caused it. If the fetus dies
more than 2 or 3 weeks after CVS, the CVS is unlikely to have caused the
death. Overall, there is a slight increase in the miscarriage rate after either
CVS or amniocentesis. It is usually recommended that you reduce your
level of activity for the 12 to 24 hours following CVS, but after this there is
no need to take extra precautions.

Which is safest—transcervical or transabdominal CVS?
There is little difference in the risks of these two techniques. The risks
depend more on the level of experience and skill of the person performing
the procedure. Ask the doctor who is to carry out your test about their
method and results.

What are the advantages and disadvantages of prenatal tests at 10–14 weeks?

The revolutionary changes in prenatal testing over the past 20 years not only
allow many abnormalities to be detected, but often they can be detected early.
For pregnant women who choose to have prenatal tests, early testing can be
very important. The time before your prenatal tests have been completed

can be very difficult and stressful. It has been described as 'the tentative pregnancy'. Should you feel excited, or is something dreadful going to be found in the tests? Should you tell family and friends? In general, women want to have these tests as early as possible, and the range of early tests now available can be of enormous psychological benefit.

Advantages of early testing

When you are only 3 months into your pregnancy, testing for chromosome abnormalities such as Down syndrome can be completed. You can choose a diagnostic test with CVS or a screening test with ultrasound, or the combined blood test and ultrasound scan. A careful ultrasound examination at 12–13 weeks can detect many of the major physical abnormalities, particularly if a vaginal scanner is used. Having completed these tests you can feel confident that unexpected abnormalities are now unlikely to be found, even at an 18–22 week scan, and that pregnancy complications such as miscarriage are unlikely.

Disadvantages of early testing

A fetus with a chromosome abnormality such as Down syndrome has a much higher chance of miscarrying than a fetus with normal chromosomes. When testing is carried out at 10–14 weeks—either by screening tests or by CVS—some Down syndrome fetuses will be detected that would have miscarried had the woman waited for later serum screening or amniocentesis. It is very distressing to have a miscarriage but the distress is even greater if tests are carried out, an abnormality found, and you choose to have an abortion.

It is more difficult for a doctor to diagnose physical abnormalities by ultrasound at 12–13 weeks than later in the pregnancy. Some abnormalities will not be picked up at the early scan. Suspected abnormalities may turn out to be fine on a later scan. If a diagnosis of an abnormality is made at an early scan, it is difficult or impossible to confirm that diagnosis after an abortion. This is because an abortion is carried out by suction curettage (see Chapter 9) and a pathological examination of the fetus is not possible.

Not all abnormalities can be detected early. Failed detection may be because the views are so technically difficult that an abnormality is missed, or because it does not develop until later in pregnancy. Late developing abnormalities include most cases of water on the brain (hydrocephaly) and many forms of dwarfism.

In reality, not all tests are available to all women at state-of-the-art level. CVS is often technically more difficult than amniocentesis and is not available at all hospitals or centers. Prenatal testing can be expensive; and not all tests are available to all women. In addition, not all hospitals have the latest technology or the expertise to examine 12–13 week fetuses carefully and provide accurate diagnosis. Some hospitals do all their scans through the abdomen and therefore detect fewer abnormalities.

No matter how good the pictures are on ultrasound at 12–13 weeks, an ultrasound examination at 18–22 weeks is recommended if you want the best check for a physical abnormality.

What are the treatment options if an abnormality is found at 10–14 weeks?

Few prenatal treatments are available at this stage, although there are some conditions where the outlook for the child is improved if the diagnosis is made before birth. Giving birth in a hospital with expert staff enables early treatment of some heart abnormalities, and sometimes the healthy survival of a baby that might have died in a less well resourced hospital. Rarely, caesarean section is recommended following the diagnosis of an abnormality, such as spina bifida.

The major decision following the diagnosis of an abnormality at 10–14 weeks is whether or not to continue the pregnancy.

If an abnormality is found and you choose to have an early termination or abortion then this can be carried out as a minor surgical procedure, a suction curette—also called a dilatation and curettage (D&C). Later abortion is not only more emotionally traumatic, but the abortion itself is a bigger procedure. It involves an induction of labor or a dilatation and evacuation (D&E) in which the much larger fetus is surgically removed from the uterus. Drugs or other methods to soften and partially dilate the cervix may precede a D&E. There are some increased risks with the later procedures. See Chapter 9 for a full description of termination procedures.

Following a later abortion there is the added problem of family and friends usually knowing about the pregnancy. This involves frequent and sometimes difficult explanations or giving some other explanation, such as having had a 'miscarriage'. The pregnancy loss is no longer a private matter and the need for explanations adds to an already devastating experience.

The main benefit of testing at this stage is to provide information to the pregnant woman to help her with her decision on whether to have a termination or to continue the pregnancy.

6 Prenatal testing: 15–17 weeks

If you have chosen to have either a blood test for Down syndrome, called mid trimester serum screening, or an amniocentesis, then these tests are carried out at this stage of pregnancy.

Ultrasound examinations are not usually done at this time—it is too late for nuchal translucency screening and too early to get the best pictures of the physical structure of your fetus. Ultrasound is used to guide the needle to the correct spot during amniocentesis, and you may be offered a scan if you develop problems such as bleeding or pain.

For most women, 15–17 weeks of pregnancy is a relaxed and healthy time. The nausea and vomiting of early pregnancy is gone, yet the fetus is still small enough not to restrict your mobility. By this stage, you will usually have resolved the often difficult decisions about which tests to have.

If you decided to have screening tests for Down syndrome, then you may already have had a nuchal translucency scan with or without a blood test (see Chapter 5, page 56). Or you may be about to have your 15–17 weeks serum screening test. If you had a nuchal translucency scan with or without serum screening, you would not usually have another blood test at 15–17 weeks unless the tests are combined to produce a single risk figure, called the integrated test. If you have two types of tests producing two separate risk figures; then you increase the chance of either one or the other test putting you in the 'increased risk' group.

If you have opted for a diagnostic test—one that provides a definitive answer on certain abnormalities—then either you will already have had chorionic villus sampling (CVS—see Chapter 5, page 63) or you will have opted for an amniocentesis at this stage. You would not usually have both amniocentesis and CVS, as they both test for the same thing—abnormalities of the chromosomes.

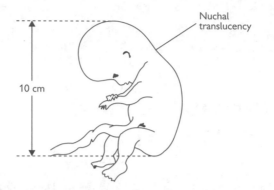

Figure 6.1 Diagram of a 15–17 week fetus

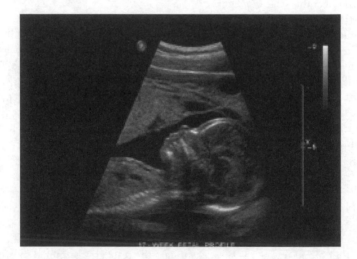

Figure 6.2 3D Image of a 15–17 week fetus

What does the fetus look like at 15–17 weeks?

The complete physical development of your fetus takes place over approximately 8 weeks and is finished by the time it is 12 weeks old. On a 12 week scan all the organs, even the fingers and toes, have developed and can usually be clearly seen. Between 12 and 40 weeks the organs are maturing so that they can work properly at birth. There is also continued rapid growth. The fetus is now about 14 cm long (crown to heel measurement), and it weighs approximately 100 grams (see Figure 6.1).

The best ultrasound views of your fetus at 15–17 weeks are usually through your abdomen. The uterus is usually too high up in the abdomen to see the fetus well with a vaginal scan. If it is lying face up and has pools of fluid around it, then beautiful ultrasound pictures can be obtained, particularly in a slim woman (see Figure 6.2).

What tests can be done at 15–17 weeks?

Serum screening (or blood tests)

Serum screening measures a combination of substances in your blood. It is often called 'mid-trimester serum screening' because the test is performed in the middle three months of pregnancy. It is also referred to as the 'double', 'triple' or 'quadruple' test depending on how many substances are tested in the pregnant woman's blood. In many regions this is the commonest test offered to pregnant women as it is low cost and convenient.

At this stage of pregnancy serum screening is an accurate test that can be used by itself, whereas early serum screening at 9–12 weeks must be done alongside nuchal translucency scanning. The major disadvantage of serum screening at 15–17 weeks is the lateness of the test.

Serum screening for Down syndrome

Serum screening provides a relatively cheap but effective method of screening for Down syndrome. The blood of a woman carrying a fetus with Down syndrome tends to contain slightly different levels of some substances that are produced by the placenta and the fetus. These include alpha fetoprotein (AFP), human chorionic gonadotrophin (HCG)—the hormone that is measured in a pregnancy test—and an oestrogen called 'unconjugated oestriol'. A combination of the age of the pregnant woman, high levels of HCG, low levels of AFP and unconjugated oestriol, may indicate an increased risk of Down syndrome. Other substances may also be included in this screening test.

A woman who is almost 37 years old has a one in 250, or more, risk of delivering a baby with Down syndrome if she does not have prenatal testing. If the result of this blood test shows your risk is higher than one in 250, you will be told you are at 'increased risk' of having a baby with Down syndrome. Approximately one in 20 pregnant women are offered an amniocentesis as a result of having had an increased risk blood test. Around 70 per cent of Down syndrome fetuses can be detected this way.

Don't forget: screening tests for Down syndrome do not detect all affected fetuses.

The older you are, the higher the chance of your serum screening result being 'increased risk'. This is because your age is used in the calculation of risk. But serum screening does not detect as high a proportion of the Down syndrome fetuses carried by younger women as it does of older women. It will detect about eight out of 10 Down syndrome fetuses in women aged 35 to 39, but only about half of those carried by women aged 25 to 29.

Only about one in 50 women identified as 'increased risk' are in fact carrying a Down syndrome fetus. If the fetus does not have Down syndrome, the increased risk serum screening result does not usually suggest any other problem. Even in a healthy pregnancy the levels of different substances in your blood vary greatly; if Down syndrome is not found at amniocentesis then an increased risk serum test result does not mean you are at increased risk of other abnormalities.

Most pregnant women with increased risk serum screening results are carrying a normal fetus, but their chance of Down syndrome is increased.

Serum screening for neural tube defects (NTDs)

NTDs are malformations of the nervous system and include spina bifida and anencephaly. In spina bifida part of the spinal column is open, often resulting in nerve damage to the legs, bladder and bowel. In anencephaly, the skull bones do not form properly, resulting in destruction of most of the brain tissue.

Alpha-fetoprotein (AFP) is a protein made by the fetus that circulates in its bloodstream to help maintain fluid balance. Tiny amounts of AFP cross into the pregnant woman's circulation causing the levels to rise in early pregnancy.

There is a high level of AFP in the fluid around the fetal spinal cord and brain; a neural tube defect causes more AFP to pass into the amniotic fluid. A higher amount also finds its way into the pregnant woman's circulation. If a high level of AFP is found in your blood at 15–17 weeks, you have an increased risk of having a baby with a neural tube defect. The AFP levels tend to be low in Down syndrome.

If you are offered serum screening for Down syndrome at 15–17 weeks, your blood will also be tested for AFP. This detects about nine out of 10 fetuses with anencephaly and eight out of 10 of those with open spina bifida. There are a small group of other abnormalities that can cause a high AFP, for example, omphalocele (also called an exomphalos) where there is a deficiency in the fetal abdominal wall.

Serum AFP is a screening test, and as such it cannot be 100 per cent accurate—it aims to select a group of fetuses for further testing. A high level of AFP is found in the blood of about one in 50 pregnant women, but only about one in 20 of these fetuses will have a neural tube defect. As NTDs can accurately be detected on a scan, an ultrasound examination is also a good screening test for identifying NTDs (see Chapter 3).

How accurate is serum screening?

An increased-risk serum screening result only occasionally means that the fetus has an abnormality, such as Down syndrome or spina bifida.

The most common causes of an increased risk result are:

(i) The pregnancy is either more or less advanced than expected—the interpretation of the result depends on the precise number of weeks of pregnancy.

(ii) There are normal variations in the level of the substances in the pregnant woman's blood.

(iii) There are twins present.

What further tests are available?

If you get an increased risk serum screening result you will be offered further tests. This will usually be an amniocentesis if there is an increased risk of Down syndrome, or ultrasound if the risk is for neural tube defects.

An ultrasound examination

This shows the age of the pregnancy and whether there is more than one fetus. If the ultrasound shows that your fetus is older or younger than you had thought, the screening test and your result may need to be reinterpreted. You may no longer be at increased risk. Ultrasound can also detect some birth defects, including all cases of anencephaly and 95 per cent of cases of spina bifida.

Amniocentesis

An amniocentesis (see page 87), or, very rarely at this stage, CVS (see Chapter 5, page 63) provides a definite answer to whether your fetus has Down syndrome or another chromosome abnormality.

How should the results of serum screening at 15–17 weeks be interpreted?

Serum screening is a complex process, and it can be difficult for couples to understand the implications of an increased risk result. Most women expect to be reassured by the test, so you may not have thought about the possibility of an increased risk result and its consequences.

Not all pregnant women want to be tested for spina bifida and Down syndrome; you should be told in advance what tests are offered and what their implications could be.

A major problem with some serum screening programs is their organization. A good laboratory service is essential as these are very sensitive tests. Unless the laboratory is well organized and does a lot of these blood tests, it may not have its normal ranges clearly enough defined to accurately report which tests are abnormal. Results are improved if an ultrasound scan is done before the blood test to assess the age of the pregnancy accurately.

Getting an 'increased risk' result is very worrying. This is partly because people are used to a medical test being either 'positive' or 'negative'; positive confirming that there is disease present, negative confirming that there is not. But serum screening is not so clear cut. Most pregnant women with an increased risk result are not carrying a fetus with Down syndrome or spina bifida. But some women with a low risk result do have a fetus with Down syndrome. Around 49 out of 50 women with an increased risk will not have a baby with Down syndrome. This is described as a false positive result.

Pregnant women who get an increased risk result often remain anxious and worried, even after an amniocentesis has shown that Down syndrome is not present. For some women, this anxiety may be based on the premise that 'there's no smoke without fire'. This logic is understandable, but incorrect. Serum screening is a test, and a relatively crude one, which indicates the risk of Down syndrome. If the serum test shows you have an increased risk, and your fetus is subsequently shown not to have the syndrome, there is usually no increased risk for the rest of your pregnancy.

A major difficulty with the 15–17 week serum screening test is that it is done at a relatively late stage of pregnancy. By the time the results of the blood tests are available, plus those of a follow-up amniocentesis if you have one, you are likely to be almost 20 weeks pregnant. Although an abortion is medically possible at any stage of pregnancy, a termination at this late stage is more emotionally traumatic. Women usually choose an earlier test, but earlier blood tests are less accurate.

Questions about serum screening at 15–18 weeks

Surely there must be something wrong if the serum screening test is abnormal?

Serum screening cannot tell you if an abnormality is present; it is a screening test which can show an increased risk of an abnormality being present.

More than 95 per cent of pregnant women who get an increased risk result have an absolutely healthy baby.

If an abnormality is causing the high or low risk result, will it always be found?

If the serum screening test shows that your fetus has an increased risk of Down syndrome, then amniocentesis will confirm whether or not the syndrome is present. If the AFP level is high, ultrasound can detect around 95 per cent of those fetuses with spina bifida. It is unlikely that a fetus with Down syndrome or spina bifida would be missed if you choose to follow up your serum screening with amniocentesis or ultrasound as appropriate.

Amniocentesis

Amniocentesis (pronounced amneo-sen-tee-sis) was the first test used to check for chromosome disorders in the fetus, and it is still the most common method used. It is a diagnostic test, that is, it can show definitely whether your fetus has a chromosomal abnormality, or whether it does not. If you are an older pregnant woman (usually defined as 35 years and above), you may be offered the option of amniocentesis or CVS (see Chapter 5, page 63).

During an amniocentesis a doctor withdraws a sample of fluid from around the developing fetus. A needle is passed through the skin of the pregnant woman, then the wall of the uterus, and is guided by ultrasound into the sac containing the amniotic fluid. This test can be carried out at any stage of pregnancy, although it is most commonly done at around 15–17 weeks.

Although women are keen to get the results as early as possible, studies have found that an earlier amniocentesis—before 15 weeks—has higher risks (see Chapter 5). It is possible to do the test later than 17 weeks, but processing the specimen may take up to two weeks, and occasionally longer, so your results would arrive late in your pregnancy.

Increasingly, pregnant women are being offered screening tests for Down syndrome. The main ones are a nuchal translucency scan at 12–13 weeks (see Chapter 5, page 56), an early blood test at 10–12 weeks (see Chapter 5, page 59) or a later one at 15–17 weeks (see page 83, this chapter). If a screening test shows an increased risk of Down syndrome, then amniocentesis is offered.

A high level of alpha-fetoprotein (AFP) is found in the amniotic fluid in spina bifida. AFP is a cheap and easy test, so it was traditionally carried out on the amniotic fluid sample, even for those at low risk. This has now largely been replaced by ultrasound.

What happens before an amniocentesis?

Most women do not find it painful, but you are likely to feel apprehensive and nervous prior to your amniocentesis, particularly if it is your first one. This anxiety should be alleviated if the procedure is explained to you. You may find it helpful to have your partner or a friend with you for support during the scan and the amniocentesis.

An ultrasound examination is done through the abdomen and is followed immediately by the amniocentesis, without you having to move from the examination couch. If you are able to relax enough to watch the TV monitor, it can be exciting to see your fetus on the ultrasound screen.

You do not need to make any special preparations for amniocentesis. If there is any doubt about how advanced your pregnancy is, your doctor may suggest you have an ultrasound scan in the weeks before the test. A full bladder is unnecessary for the ultrasound examination or the amniocentesis, although your doctor might ask you not to pass urine in the hour before the test.

You should know your blood group before an amniocentesis. Any procedure that involves passing a needle into the uterus can result in some blood cells from the fetus crossing into the circulation of the pregnant woman. If you are one of the 15 per cent of people who have Rhesus negative blood, fetal cells may cause you to develop antibodies to clear your circulation of these 'foreign' cells. These antibodies in turn cross the placenta. The level of antibody may rise in subsequent pregnancies and destroy enough of the red cells in the fetal circulation to cause it to become anaemic. This is called Rhesus (Rh) disease. To prevent a Rhesus negative pregnant woman making these antibodies, an injection called 'anti-D' (or Rhogam in the USA) may be given to destroy the fetal red blood cells. A blood sample is usually taken before the injection is given, to ensure that antibodies are not already present.

What happens during an amniocentesis?

An area on your abdomen is prepared by cleaning your skin with antiseptic solution. A local anesthetic is not used because amniocentesis is a relatively painless procedure. The ultrasound pad, or transducer, is placed on your skin and moved around until it locates an area where the needle can be inserted straight into the amniotic fluid, without making contact with your fetus. If possible the placenta is also avoided. The needle is plunged rapidly through the skin, down to the right depth. See Figure 6.3. The doctor watches the needle on the ultrasound screen from the moment it enters the skin until it is withdrawn, and so is able to adjust its position to avoid your fetus.

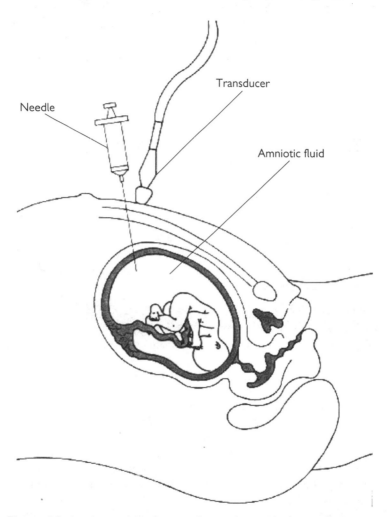

Needle

Transducer

Amniotic fluid

Figure 6.3 Amniocentesis: ultrasound is used to guide the needle into a pocket of fluid

Some doctors pass the needle through a frame attached to the side of the ultrasound transducer. Once the needle tip is in the right place, a syringe is attached and the amniotic fluid is drawn up. The first 1 or 2 ml may be discarded, as it may contain cells collected from the pregnant woman's tissues. 15 ml of fluid, about 3 teaspoons, is withdrawn, the needle is removed, and the heartbeat of the fetus is re-checked. It is extremely rare to find any irregularity of the heartbeat after the test.

The doctor doing your amniocentesis should be experienced in performing the technique under ultrasound guidance. It is reasonable to expect your doctor to be doing at least 50 amniocenteses each year. In general, the test is safer when it is carried out by a doctor who does a lot of them.

After your amniocentesis, you will probably be advised to sit down and wait for a short time before you leave. You should be capable of driving yourself home, but you might appreciate having somebody with you, as you may feel tired and emotionally drained afterwards. Many women have been psychologically preparing for the amniocentesis for some time. It is a good idea to relax at home for the rest of the day, although there should be no reason to go to bed. Occasionally the needle may puncture a small blood vessel under your skin resulting in a bruise and minor discomfort. Most doctors say you can return to normal activities the day after your test and for the rest of the pregnancy.

Is an amniocentesis painful?

For most women, amniocentesis is a psychologically stressful experience, and a focus for all their fears about abnormalities. Women's experiences of physical pain vary. Amniocentesis performed by an experienced doctor does not usually cause you more than mild discomfort. To many women it is no more painful than a blood test.

Experienced operators can almost always pass the needle into the amniotic fluid on the first attempt. A very fine needle is used (usually 22 gauge), which minimizes the risks and causes the least distress. Because most women dread the procedure, they are usually surprised that a needle can be passed into their uterus with minimal discomfort.

A sample of women in Melbourne, Australia, were asked to fill out a questionnaire after amniocentesis. 83 per cent said the test was less painful than they had expected. 86 per cent said it caused no discomfort or only mild discomfort, while 14 per cent said it had caused them some pain.

I had read enough about amniocentesis to think that it would be awful. My husband came along and we had both built up a lot of apprehension. But I was lucky. The gynaecologist was terrific, probably the best around. It was definitely uncomfortable seeing the needle go into my abdomen, but it was not painful. I was distracted by the procedure, so the ultrasound examination of the fetus had little impact. We had been ambivalent about having children, but my husband fell in love with our son when he saw him on the ultrasound screen.

A local anaesthetic can be used to desensitize the skin, although most doctors do not encourage this. This solution of local anaesthetic requires an injection which stings as it goes in, and a second needle must then be inserted for the amniocentesis. Most women feel that the pain of the anaesthetic injection is worse than the passage of the needle without it.

What are the risks of amniocentesis?

Miscarriage

The most drastic and the most feared risk of amniocentesis is miscarriage. Many studies have been done to assess this risk, but it is difficult to put a precise figure on the likelihood of miscarriage as a result of an amniocentesis. Different doctors use slightly different techniques, which may result in different complication rates. It is often impossible to tell if a miscarriage after amniocentesis is due to the procedure, or if it would have happened anyway. It is likely that a miscarriage the day after amniocentesis was due to the test and that one four weeks later was not, but it is impossible to be sure.

Without amniocentesis, about 0.7 per cent of pregnancies that appear normal on ultrasound at 16 weeks will subsequently miscarry. This is called the 'background' rate, but it is not a precise figure. To find out how many pregnancies miscarry after amniocentesis, the background rate is subtracted from the total number that miscarry. This gives an approximate measure of the increased risk of miscarriage due to the test. The best estimate is that amniocentesis increases your risk of miscarriage by about one in 200. The risk is higher if the test is carried out before 15 weeks of pregnancy.

By the age of 35 years, your numerical risk of Down syndrome being detected at amniocentesis is one in 280. This is close to the risk of miscarriage from amniocentesis, which is about one in 200. This is a difficult comparison to make. Risks are perceived differently by different women, depending on their attitudes towards disabilities and their childbearing history.

Other complications of amniocentesis

Many women fear that the needle may hit their fetus. This can nearly always be avoided, as the needle is constantly watched via ultrasound on the television monitor. If the fetus comes near, the needle can usually be moved to avoid it. Even if the needle does go into the fetus, it will cause no more harm than having a needle passed into the same place on your own body. Some fetuses that have undergone procedures such as a blood transfusions may have needles stuck into them a dozen times, usually without a single mark being visible on their skin after birth.

One large study suggested that amniocentesis increases the chances of a baby being born with club feet or dislocated hips. Other studies have not confirmed this, so it is unlikely that the risk of these abnormalities is increased by amniocentesis.

Several studies have suggested that amniocentesis causes a slight increase—about six in 1000—in the risk of breathing disorders immediately after birth, particularly in babies born between 34 and 37 weeks. The reason for this increase is unknown, and it has not been proved to be a complication of amniocentesis. One suggestion is that it is related to the amount of fluid taken during the test. For this reason it is recommended that no more fluid than necessary should be removed during amniocentesis.

Amniotic fluid leaks from the vagina after about one in 100 amniocenteses—presumably through a hole in the membranes. This is more common if amniocentesis is carried out before 15 weeks. When this happens there is a small gush of clear fluid from the vagina, within 24 hours of the test. It usually lasts only a short time or is a single gush. This fluid loss usually settles rapidly, and the pregnancy continues normally. Only rarely does the fluid loss continue, causing miscarriage or other problems.

If you have abdominal pain, or if you lose water or blood through the vagina, you should report it to your doctor who will usually advise bed rest. These symptoms should settle down. Usually you will not miscarry.

The risks of amniocentesis to you, the pregnant woman, are extremely low. Theoretically, passing a 'foreign body' or needle, into the uterus could cause infection, but this has rarely been reported. One study showed that generalized infection occurred in only one of 7579 patients. The risk of Rhesus negative women developing antibodies after amniocentesis is very low (see page 88).

Passing a needle straight into the amniotic fluid can cause blood staining of the specimen, but this is very rare. One series of 500 women was tested without a single specimen being stained. Blood staining tends to happen if there are technical difficulties during amniocentesis. It has been suggested that if blood staining occurs there is a two or three-fold increase in the risk of miscarriage, but even then the risk is quite low. Sometimes the amniotic fluid is brown due to old blood which had accumulated at the time of an earlier threatened miscarriage. This may still indicate a slight increase in the risk of miscarriage, not because of the amniocentesis, but because of the earlier bleeding. Bleeding in pregnancy means an increased risk of miscarriage.

Studies have shown that multiple needle insertions increase the miscarriage rate following the test, and that the risk increases with each needle attempt.

Two insertions of the needle are required in 2 to 3 per cent of amniocenteses. Some studies have also suggested an increased risk if the needle passes through the placenta, although others have found no such increase. It is reasonable to expect that the increased risk would depend on how thick a portion of the placenta was traversed. If care is taken to pass through a thin portion, any increase in risk is likely to be minimal.

What happens to the sample?

Your specimen of amniotic fluid is sent to a laboratory where it is processed. It is put into a centrifuge, which spins all the cells to the bottom of a tube. The cells at the bottom of the tube are placed in a culture dish or bottle with culture medium. This is then put into an incubator and the cells are allowed to grow. These cells come from the fetus's skin, connective tissue, lining of respiratory, alimentary and urinary tracts and from the amniotic membranes.

This cell growth can take anything from a few days to occasionally as long as 3 weeks. When adequate numbers of colonies or cells have grown, the specimen is taken out of the incubator and carefully examined. At least 15 cells are usually analyzed. The chromosomes are counted to ensure that there are 46, and they are individually examined to make sure the structure and banding of each appears normal. This is a lengthy process requiring highly skilled personnel. A digital photograph is taken of the chromosomes from one or two cells. Each chromosome is then cut out, paired with its opposite member and placed in numerical sequence using an image analysis system and special software.

When do I get my results?

Waiting for the result of an amniocentesis can be the most difficult part of the process for many women. It may take up to 2 weeks for you to receive the full results, although FISH and PCR results (see below) are usually back within 48 hours. These times vary because laboratory techniques differ. Even within one laboratory, reporting times vary with the speed of growth of the cells and the workload. No matter how small your chance of an abnormal result, your attention is likely to be focused on waiting for the result of your amniocentesis.

Testing with FISH and PCR

FISH (fluorescence in situ hybridization) and PCR (polymerase chain reaction) are DNA tests. These techniques are a very quick way to test for the most common chromosome abnormalities because they can be performed directly on the specimen without the need for lengthy cell culture. Results are usually available within 24–48 hours.

FISH works by using a coloured fluorescent label that attaches to a specific piece of chromosomal DNA within the cell. Cells from a person with normal chromosomes will show two fluorescent spots within each cell that represent the pair of chromosomes being tested. An individual with Down syndrome will show three fluorescent spots because there are three copies of chromosome 21 instead of the usual two. The most common FISH test uses 5 different labels and can exclude about 90 per cent of significant chromosome abnormalities by testing for chromosome 21, as well as trisomy 13 and 18 and the loss or gain of the sex chromosomes (chromosomes X and Y). Because of the cost involved, FISH is only used to test for these major abnormalities unless there is a special reason to test for something else.

PCR is an alternative method of rapidly testing for common chromosome abnormalities in amniocentesis and CVS specimens. The PCR test works by isolating and then multiplying very small amounts of DNA that has been extracted from the cells. This amplified DNA is then tested on a special machine that checks the number of chromosomes present. Both FISH and PCR are very efficient at quickly screening for the common chromosome abnormalities and the choice of test usually rests with the preference and expertise of the testing laboratory. PCR is more amenable to large scale testing and is therefore more common in larger, centralised laboratories.

It is important to realize that FISH and PCR only test for a specific group of chromosome abnormalities—the most common ones. The traditional culture method described earlier in this chapter, is always done as well as FISH, since this allows every chromosome to be fully analysed.

DNA testing is also available to couples whose pregnancy is at risk of a specific gene defect. These include cystic fibrosis and fragile X syndrome. Many other diseases can be tested for, and this number increases each year. Each disease tested is expensive; so these tests are not usually offered unless there is a specific reason to do so. The most common reason is that the couple or a close relative already has a child affected by the disease.

Does an amniocentesis always produce a result?

Amniocentesis has now been refined to such a stage that once you have decided to have the test, you can be almost sure it will be successful. However, even in the most experienced hands a test may fail. Less than 1 per cent of women need a repeat test, either because insufficient fluid is obtained or because of problems with the laboratory culture. Technical difficulties are uncommon during an amniocentesis, except, rarely, where there is very little fluid around the fetus. Occasionally, the laboratory may receive a good specimen, but for some inexplicable reason none of the cells grow and so cannot be analyzed. One reason for failed growth is that bacteria somehow get into the specimen. The laboratory can have difficulty if the specimen is very blood stained.

Amniocentesis in multiple pregnancies

About two thirds of twin pregnancies are non-identical twins. Each non-identical twin has a risk of abnormality similar to that of a single fetus. Therefore, if you are pregnant with twins, there is mostly double the risk of one of your fetuses having an abnormality compared to someone with a single fetus. With triplets the risk increases threefold, and so on. In a multiple pregnancy, amniocentesis is offered for the same reasons as in a single pregnancy, if there are risk factors such as your age. Since two insertions of the needle are necessary with twins, there is likely to be an increased risk. Results vary, but it is suggested that the risk of miscarriage is around 1 per cent or 1 in 100.

There is usually no problem sampling the fluid in the sac around each of the fetuses to test them individually. The doctor carefully searches for the membrane between the two fetuses and makes sure that fluid is taken from each sac in turn, usually by passing a needle through the skin at two separate sites. After taking the first specimen, a dye may be injected into the fluid, to ensure it is not sampled again. Some doctors believe this dye is unnecessary.

Questions about amniocentesis at 15–17 weeks

How long does the needle stay inside me?

It takes about 60 seconds for the doctor to insert the needle through the skin, withdraw the amniotic fluid and remove it. The needle does not have to be moved once it is placed in the fluid, so it does not hurt as the fluid is being withdrawn. You will have no 'pulling' inside and no other feelings as the fluid is removed from your uterus.

Is it possible that my cells will grow in the laboratory instead of those of the fetus?

This is called 'contamination' of the specimen with your cells. The methods described in this chapter are now so reliable that it is very rare indeed for maternal contamination to occur.

If amniocentesis causes a miscarriage, when would this happen?
Unfortunately there is no simple answer to this question. There is no way of telling whether a miscarriage after amniocentesis is due to the amniocentesis or would have happened anyway. Miscarriages can occur at any stage in pregnancy, whether or not you have an amniocentesis, so there is no time when you are totally 'safe'. In general it is assumed that miscarriages in the few weeks after amniocentesis are more likely to be due to the test, whereas those that occur much later, are likely to be unrelated.

Why is the fluid yellow?
When red blood cells are broken down in the fetus, a yellow substance called bilirubin is produced. The bilirubin tends to accumulate in the amniotic fluid in early pregnancy and gives it the yellow color, which is quite normal. As pregnancy advances the fluid tends to become clearer.

How do you make sure the needle will not touch the fetus?
Theoretically the doctor could go off course during amniocentesis and touch the fetus. Or, the fetus could move into the path of the needle. However, as long as the doctor watches the needle on the TV monitor, these situations are usually easily avoided. Even if the fetus does come into contact with the needle, it should not be harmed.

How much fluid does the doctor take?
Usually about 15 ml, which is less than 10 per cent of the amount of fluid present at 16 weeks.

How long does it take for the fluid to be replaced?
The fetus continuously produces and removes the fluid around itself. By the end of pregnancy more than a litre of amniotic fluid is produced daily and the same amount removed. It is hard to tell how long it takes for the total amount of fluid to return to what it was before the amniocentesis, but it presumably takes several days.

Won't the fluid leak out of the hole in my skin?
The needle used is so fine that the hole closes off immediately and fluid does not come out through the skin afterwards.

Can amniocentesis tell the sex of the fetus?
Analysis of the chromosomes automatically indicates the sex. Your doctor can tell you the sex if you wish to know.

Is it true that I must have an amniocentesis if I'm over 37?
Amniocentesis is an option available to couples who are seeking prenatal diagnosis. There should never be any compulsion to have the test. You will

be given advice and information, but ultimately you are free to make your own decision.

Ultrasound

Ultrasound scans are not usually done at 15–17 weeks. However ultrasound may be used for one of the following reasons:

1. Ultrasound is used before the amniocentesis to check the pregnancy and during the amniocentesis to guide the needle.

2. If the serum screening result shows an increased risk of a neural tube defect, ultrasound is used to check the spine, head, and the fetus in general. Although most neural tube defects can be seen on ultrasound at 15–17 weeks, a further scan at around 20 weeks can check for abnormalities when the fetus is larger.

3. Follow up of a possible abnormality seen on an earlier scan—the amount of detailed information about the fetal structure seen on ultrasound increases with each passing week from 10 weeks to 20 weeks. If the findings of an earlier scan, for example, a 12 week nuchal translucency scan, raised the suspicion of an abnormality, a repeat scan may be suggested at 15–17 weeks.

4. Other reasons for an ultrasound scan at 15–17 weeks include complications of pregnancy such as pain or bleeding.

Screening tests For Down syndrome

TEST	Results back at approximately	Approx detection rate	Other benefits	COST
NT	12–13 wks	70%	Twins/NTD and many other FA	+ +
NT + MSS T1	12–13 wks	90%		+ + +
NT + MSS T2	16–17 wks	? 95%	NTD	+ + +
T2 MSS	16–17 wks	70%	NTD	+

NT—Nuchal translucency
MSS—maternal serum screening
T1—First trimester (first 3 months)
T2—Second trimester (second 3 months)
FA—Fetal abnormality
NTD—Neural tube defect

Diagnostic tests for chromosome abnormality

TEST	TIMING (Weeks)	RISK (%)
Early amniocentesis	12–14	? 2
Amniocentesis	15+	½ (maximum)
CVS	10+	1 (maximum)

Advantages and disadvantages of prenatal tests at 15–17 weeks

Amniocentesis

The main advantage of amniocentesis is that it is the most widely available test that provides certainty about each of your fetus's chromosomes. The test is at least as safe as CVS.

The major disadvantage of amniocentesis is that it is safest if performed at 15 weeks or later—so you get your results late in your pregnancy.

Serum screening

A serum screening result at 15–17 weeks is accurate enough to be used on its own. Early serum screening at 10–12 weeks must be combined with a nuchal translucency measurement. As with amniocentesis, the major disadvantage of serum screening at 15–17 weeks is the lateness of the test.

Ultrasound

In general terms, the ultrasound images improve with each passing week of pregnancy until around 25 weeks. A scan at 15–17 weeks will provide better images and clearer diagnoses than a 12–14 week scan, but not as clear as an 18–22 week scan. Scans at this time are therefore carried out only for special reasons.

What are the treatment options at 15–17 weeks?

If an increased risk result is found following serum screening at 15–17 weeks of pregnancy, you will be offered further tests. An 'increased risk' result does not mean there is a problem. These further tests are either an amniocentesis, if there is an increased risk of Down syndrome, or an ultrasound examination if there is an increased risk of a neural tube defect.

Occasionally an ultrasound examination at 15–17 weeks raises the suspicion of an abnormality, but it is too early to be certain. In that case the scan is repeated, usually some time between 18 and 22 weeks. If there is uncertainty, you are bound to be anxious and want a quick answer. It can be very stressful waiting, often for several weeks, to find out if there is an abnormality or not.

Termination of pregnancy

See Chapter 9 for details of termination procedures.

From a medical viewpoint, a termination of pregnancy, or an abortion, can now be carried out safely at any time of pregnancy. Local laws, however, restrict how late a termination may be performed. One of the major disadvantages of amniocentesis is that if you choose to have an abortion following abnormal results, you will be between 17 and 20 weeks pregnant. Most doctors will recommend inducing labor at this stage, although some clinics offer a surgical abortion, called a dilatation and evacuation (D&E). While complications following an abortion are uncommon at any time, the risks are slightly higher at this late stage.

Dilatation and evacuation is performed under general anaesthesic. It involves dilating the cervix and removing the pregnancy with forceps, so the pregnant woman does not have to go through labor. Some drugs may be given before D&E to soften the cervix so it is easier to dilate.

To induce labor, a substance called prostaglandin, is usually placed in the vagina, to start uterine contractions. It takes between 12 and 24 hours from that time until delivery, although most of this time is spent waiting for the contractions to start. During labor, pain relief can be given if necessary, using pethidine or an epidural anaesthetic.

Deciding to have an abortion is a terribly difficult decision, even it is early in your pregnancy, and even if a major abnormality has been found. It is even more difficult if your partner is not in absolute agreement with you about what to do. Suddenly you are both forced to consider fundamental issues—is it OK to have an abortion? Is this abnormality 'severe enough' to warrant an abortion? Often, there are uncertainties about how severely the abnormality will affect the child's life. How can you weigh this up? While you can ask friends and professionals what they would do, that does not tell you what is right for you. You, your partner, and the other siblings, are the ones who will live with the decision. It is worth considering carefully whose advice you will seek—most people have a clear idea how others should run their lives. The more people you ask the more confusing it might become. We recommend that you have discussions with your doctor, midwife and other professionals he or she might recommend, along with carefully selected family and/or friends.

If the decision must be delayed until 20 weeks, and you are already feeling movements, then your choices are even harder. There can be no denying that an abortion is likely to be psychologically traumatic. Women in this situation need plenty of family support and may wish to consider professional counseling.

Termination when there is a multiple pregnancy

If you have a multiple pregnancy and an abnormality is found, it usually affects just one fetus (unless they are identical twins). In this situation three options are available. You may wish to continue, knowing one fetus has an abnormality, but being prepared to accept that outcome. Or, you could terminate the pregnancy with both fetuses being aborted together. Finally, there is the option known as selective abortion, which involves injecting a solution of a potassium salt into the heart of the fetus with the abnormality, causing it to die quickly. The risk to the surviving fetus (or fetuses) is low. The dead fetus stays inside your uterus and is delivered at the end of the pregnancy, without affecting the growth or well-being of the live fetus (or fetuses). Most couples in this situation choose selective abortion rather than aborting both fetuses.

Selective abortion is not carried out if it appears that the fetuses are monochorionic; that is, identical twins coming from one egg with one placenta, because then their circulations mix at the placenta and the death of one could affect the surviving identical twin. Fortunately, most twin pregnancies where there is one fetus with an abnormality are dichorionic; that is, non-identical, with two separate placental circulations.

If you know that you would wish to continue with the pregnancy even if an abnormality was found in one fetus, then you might consider not having amniocentesis.

7 Prenatal testing: 18–22 weeks

You are now approximately half way through your pregnancy. You will soon be able to feel your fetus move, or you may already have felt it. It is time for your last prenatal test—the 'routine' mid trimester ultrasound examination. This scan is much awaited, often a family event, and a major photo opportunity. But don't forget that it is an important medical examination for your fetus.

Within 30 years ultrasound has developed from primitive black and white images giving only the most basic information, to sophisticated images showing exquisite detail of the physical structure of a fetus. With improvements in ultrasound technology a whole new discipline of medicine has emerged, that of prenatal diagnosis. Almost all prenatal tests require ultrasound either to make the diagnosis or to guide the taking of a specimen.

A wide range of abnormalities can be detected on ultrasound. Some are so serious that they result in death during pregnancy or shortly after birth, others are simply 'markers' of a possible problem, particularly of chromosome abnormality. Markers are not abnormalities, as they cause no problems themselves, but they are variations in the appearance of structures, that are sometimes linked to a problem after birth. The commonest markers are those for Down syndrome. One example is echogenic bowel—the intestines in the fetal abdomen look brighter than usual. Markers are described in detail later in this chapter (see page 119).

The ultrasound scan at 18–22 weeks is the last, but psychologically often the biggest hurdle of all the prenatal tests. It is important, as it brings home to many women the reality of their pregnancy. You can actually see your fetus on the screen, often for the first time. If the scan is fine, you can expect the baby to arrive in around 20 weeks time and you should have a high degree of confidence that he or she will be healthy. But remember that prenatal tests cannot guarantee a healthy baby. Sometimes abnormalities are missed, and many abnormalities are not usually tested for. Others cannot be detected, and some develop late in pregnancy.

Don't be fooled by the 'routine' aspect of this test. This mid pregnancy scan is a prenatal test, and it is your choice whether to have prenatal testing. You can decide whether or not you want this examination. You might decide that you only wish to know about abnormalities of a certain severity. It has been suggested that women should be given the opportunity of choosing what level of information they wish to receive—you need to say in advance if you don't want to have some minor abnormalities or 'markers' reported to you.

How can I make the most of my ultrasound examination?

This scan is a wonderful, often emotional, experience and one to be enjoyed and savoured. There are things that you can do to try to ensure that you have the best possible experience and the most effective examination.

Take the person or people you wish to share the experience with you. If this includes children, ensure that there is an adult present to care for each child, and that the adult is happy to leave with the child if and when they get restless. Crying and restless children are a distraction for many scan operators and can affect their concentration. The other thing you can do is make sure you have the scan at the right time. While excellent pictures can be obtained at 18 weeks in slim women, much better pictures are obtained at 20 weeks in women who are overweight.

You can make sure you get the best possible ultrasound examination by asking questions. These questions could be answered either by your referring doctor or midwife, or by the hospital or centre where the examination is planned:

1. Qualifications: What are the ultrasound qualifications available and does the doctor who will be responsible for your examination have it or them?

2. How many pregnancy scans does he or she carry out on average a day? If the answer is more than 10, then they are committed to this work.

3. Where would your doctor, your doctor's wife, or your midwife go for their own pregnancy scan?

4. Is the equipment that will be used for your scan a top of the range machine?

5. If a sonographer or technician is doing your scan, how experienced is he or she and how many pregnancy scans do they do on average a day?

What does the fetus look like at 18–22 weeks?

Your fetus has been fully developed from 12 weeks of pregnancy, with all of its arms, legs, and internal organs formed. Since then it has simply been growing, and the organs have been maturing. Your fetus will have been moving since you were 8 weeks pregnant, although most women don't feel movements until around 20 weeks. Some women feel them much earlier than this, particularly if they have had other children. By 18–22 weeks your fetus is around 23 cm long and weighs about 400 g, or nearly 1 lb (see Figure 7.1). It is now big enough to be able to see most of its physical structures with ultrasound. While beautiful views of structures can be obtained earlier in pregnancy, many of these can be seen in more detail now.

What tests can be done at 18–22 weeks?

The only test that is usually done at this stage of pregnancy is an ultrasound examination—18–22 weeks is usually considered the best time for looking at fetal development. Some abnormalities, such as heart problems, are often not evident until this stage of pregnancy. Some other abnormalities do not even develop until this stage, including some cases of hydrocephaly (water in the brain), microcephaly (small head), hydronephrosis (blocked kidneys), and dwarfism.

By 18–22 weeks most of the abnormalities that can be detected by ultrasound can be seen, and it is still possible to have an abortion, if this is what you want, in most legal systems. The time that is chosen for your scan

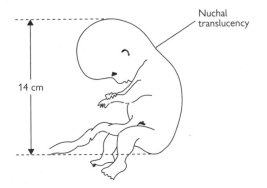

Figure 7.1 Diagram of an 18 week fetus

varies to some extent with the law on abortion. If abortion is only available before 20 weeks of pregnancy, then scans are usually done at 18 weeks, so that your decision can be made by 20 weeks. If abortion is available later, some centers will suggest delaying the scan until 20 or even 22 weeks.

What is the 18–22 week ultrasound examination for?

One of the wonderful things about ultrasound is that it allows women and their loved ones to bond with their developing baby. But this is not the top priority for this important medical examination. There are many reasons for having an ultrasound examination at 18–22 weeks, but the focus of the examination is to check the physical structure of your fetus for possible abnormalities. See pages 109–119 for details of the structural abnormalities that ultrasound can detect.

Although it is a medical examination, it can be a social event too. Seeing clear pictures of your fetus is a unique experience that you and your partner should enjoy. Photos will be offered, and it may be possible to take a video or DVD home. Images are now being offered on CD Rom, or in other ways, so that they can be emailed to friends. The sex can be identified at this scan. Ask, if you want to know.

As well as checking the physical structure of your fetus, the purpose of an ultrasound scan is:

To check the age of your fetus and how it is growing

The first scan in pregnancy is the most accurate time to date a pregnancy, as early on your fetus grows at a very rapid and a very constant rate. If you did not have an earlier scan, then your dates are confirmed with this scan. If you did have an earlier scan, this scan checks that growth has been normal. It will not reconsider your dates unless there has been an error in the measurements on your first scan. The age of your pregnancy and predicting your due date are discussed in Chapter 4.

To discover if it is a single or a multiple pregnancy

Ultrasound can identify the number of fetuses present, as each heartbeat and each amniotic sac can be seen. Multiple pregnancies are rarely missed as a scan provides a section or slice all the way through the pregnancy. The fetuses cannot hide behind one another and avoid being seen. See Chapter 4 for details of early ultrasound and multiple pregnancies.

To find out the position of the placenta

An 18–22 week scan is a screening test for a low-lying placenta. In the first 8 weeks of pregnancy, the placenta, then called the chorion, surrounds all of the developing fetus and its pregnancy sac. From 9 weeks, this begins to thicken around one side of the pregnancy sac to form the placenta, and it thins around the rest of the pregnancy sac. As the fetus grows, the placenta occupies a smaller proportion of the wall of the uterus. By 18 weeks it occupies about one third of the wall of the uterus and by the time of birth, about one sixth of the wall of the uterus. When a scan is carried out at 18 weeks, the placenta will often appear to be low-lying, but this often changes by the end of the pregnancy. The placenta looks low in up to one in 20 pregnancies at 18 weeks, but for most of these women, the placenta will not be low at the time of delivery. 'Placenta praevia' actually occurs in about one in 200 pregnancies. By carefully examining the exact position of the placenta, a skilled operator can estimate the chance of the placenta being low at the time of delivery.

If you are told that your placenta is low-lying at 18 weeks, don't let this worry you. It simply means that a further scan should be done later in pregnancy, at around 32 weeks, to determine the ultimate position of your placenta. In the meantime there is no need to alter your activities or lifestyle in any way, unless your doctor advises you to do so.

Other checks

These include checking the amount of amniotic fluid, whether there is an ovarian cyst, or fibroids—thickenings in the muscle wall of the uterus—and the length of the cervix. The position of the umbilical cord can also be seen. It is often around the neck of the fetus, but this only causes problems at delivery if it is tightly wrapped.

See pages 109–119 for details of specific structural abnormalities that can be detected by ultrasound at this stage of pregnancy.

Don't forget, magnificent modern ultrasound technology does not guarantee a normal baby. Ultrasound allows many physical handicaps to be detected, but it does not even guarantee that the fetus's structure is normal.

How is an ultrasound scan done?

An ultrasound scan involves high frequency sound waves being passed into your body. The reflected echoes are then analyzed to build up a picture of the fetus in your uterus. Two dimensional (2D) ultrasound is normally used. This takes 'slices' through tissues and analyzes the cut slices or cross sections. The pregnancy is carefully and systematically examined by the scan operator. This examination can diagnose many different abnormalities, and it gives most couples great reassurance that their fetus is likely to be born without a problem.

What is 3D and 4D ultrasound?

3D and 4D ultrasound are the latest in a long line of major breakthroughs over the past 30 years. They have grabbed public attention because of the life-like moving images that can be obtained, providing excitement for the pregnant woman and her partner and bonding with the child to be.

3D can show life-like images (see Figure 7.2) and 4D, which is a moving 3D image, can show the fetus waving its arms and kicking. Comments such as 'That's amazing', 'I can't believe you can see that', 'That's fantastic' are common. But also quite common is 'It looks like an alien', or 'I can't see that'. Many 3D and 4D pictures can be poor or make the fetus look abnormal.

The best 3D and 4D is available with new and expensive state of the art equipment. Since most diagnoses do not need 3D and ultrasound is primarily a medical service, most machines in use do not have the best 3D. Usually the medical examination is carried out with 2D and if 3D is used, it is at the end to produce some family snaps. The quality of 3D and 4D

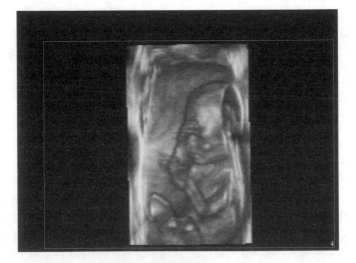

Figure 7.2 3D image of an 18–20 week fetus

pictures very much depends however on how clear the 2D pictures are. These vary with which way the fetus is facing, the weight of the pregnant woman, and other factors. The general rule is, if the 2D pictures are not very good, the 3D pictures are poor.

3D and 4D ultrasound can enhance the pregnancy experience, but most centres find that 2D is usually still best for diagnosis. It may not yet be available in your area. Increasingly however, 3D is being used for assessing some abnormalities. Because it can be used for looking at surface layers, 3D is good for looking for the face and assessing abnormalities such as a cleft or hare lip. Another advantage of 3D ultrasound is that after the patient has left the room, slices can be made through stored volumes of tissues—this is not done at the moment.

The American Institute of Ultrasound in Medicine summed up the new technology as follows:

'Currently, two-dimensional (2D) gray-scale real-time sonography is the primary method of medically indicated anatomic imaging with ultrasound. While three dimensional (3D) sonography may be helpful in diagnosis, it should not be considered more than a developing technology. Its role is restricted to an adjunct of, but not a replacement for, 2D ultrasound. As with any developing technology, its diagnostic value may improve, and its diagnostic role will be periodically re-evaluated. This will change, however, but few practices today use 3D in a major way to make diagnoses.'

Don't be disappointed if the ultrasound machine does not have 3D or 4D, or the images are indecipherable to you because your fetus is facing away. The important thing is that the scan operator is doing their job thoroughly. Missing a photo opportunity is better than a missed diagnosis at a vital medical examination!

What are the risks of ultrasound scans?

Some women are concerned about the effect of ultrasound on their developing baby, and there have been regular ultrasound 'scares' over the years. One finding has been of a higher chance of left handedness in boys following prenatal ultrasound.

The developing fetus is sensitive to external agents, particularly in the first 3 months of pregnancy. Some techniques may use a higher level of ultrasound, such as pulsed Doppler, that traces the blood flow. These higher power levels, like Doppler, are not usually used in early pregnancy. If you can hear the heartbeat of your fetus, or what sounds like it, during an ultrasound examination, then pulsed Doppler is being used.

There is no conclusive research evidence of serious adverse health effects from prenatal ultrasound exposure, but the evidence is incomplete.

In summary, ultrasound is considered safe when it is used for medical purposes. All professional bodies discourage what might be called the frivolous uses of ultrasound, or using ultrasound for social purposes alone, with no medical benefit.

To improve the quality of pictures, there is a tendency for manufacturers to increase power levels in ultrasound equipment. In addition, the American Food and Drug Administration (FDA) has relaxed the restrictions on the power levels that can be used in obstetric examinations, relying on the operator to limit the exposure by noting power levels that are registered on the screen.

The following statements from a range of international bodies advocate a cautious and vigilant approach to ultrasound.

'Ultrasound is now accepted as being of considerable diagnostic value. There is no evidence that diagnostic ultrasound has produced any harm to patients in the four decades that it has been in use. However, the acoustic output of modern equipment is generally much greater than that of the early equipment and, in view of the continuing progress in equipment design and applications, outputs may be expected to continue to be subject to change. Also, investigations into the possibility of subtle or transient effects are still in an early stage. Consequently diagnostic ultrasound can only be considered safe if used prudently.' (Safety Group of the British Medical Ultrasound Society).

The following is taken from the Safety Statement, 2000 (reconfirmed 2003) of the International Society of Ultrasound in Obstetrics and Gynecology (ISUOG). 'Based on evidence currently available, routine clinical scanning of every woman during pregnancy using real time B-mode imaging is not contraindicated. The risk of damage to the fetus by teratogenic agents is particularly great in the first trimester. One has to remember that heat is generated at the transducer surface when using the transvaginal approach. Spectral and colour Doppler may produce high intensities, and routine examination by this modality during the embryonic period is rarely indicated. In addition, because of high acoustic absorption by bone, the potential for heating adjacent tissues must also be kept in mind.

Exposure time and acoustic output should be kept to the lowest levels consistent with obtaining diagnostic information and limited to medically indicated procedures, rather than for purely entertainment purposes.'

'The American Institute of Ultrasound in Medicine (AIUM) advocates the responsible use of diagnostic ultrasound. The AIUM strongly discourages the non-medical use of ultrasound for psychosocial or entertainment purposes. The use of either two dimensional (2D) or three dimensional (3D) ultrasound to only view the fetus, obtain a picture of the fetus or determine the fetal gender without a medical indication is inappropriate and contrary to responsible medical practice. Although there are no confirmed biological effects on patients caused by exposures from present diagnostic ultrasound instruments, the possibility exists that such biological effects may be identified in the future. Thus ultrasound should be used in a prudent manner to provide medical benefit to the patient.' (American Institute of Ultrasound in Medicine).

What structural abnormalities can be detected by ultrasound at 18–22 weeks?

Ultrasound produces a series of sections, usually cross sections, through the fetus to check the structures and organs. The detail that can be seen could fill a whole textbook. Below are some of the important structures that can be examined and some of the abnormalities that can be seen. See Chapter 2 for details of fetal abnormalities.

Head and spine

Figure 7.3 shows a section high up in the head with the skull encasing the brain. It is not a view from above the head, but a slice through the tissues of the skull and brain, so that the structure of the brain itself can be seen. This section is carefully examined as it contains the midline between the two hemispheres of the brain, as well as the lateral ventricles, which are the main fluid-containing chambers. Three important abnormalities can be detected using this section.

Anencephaly is a condition in which the bony skull and most of the brain is absent. It is easily identified, as the structures normally seen in this section through the head and brain are all missing. There is no treatment, and the baby dies before or immediately after birth. The incidence of anencephaly varies from between 0.5 and 2 births per 1000. It is most common in Ireland and Wales, and uncommon in Asian countries.

Hydrocephaly is an increase in the amount of cerebrospinal fluid in the chambers of the brain. It happens in 0.5 to 3 births per 1000, and it is diagnosed when the size of the ventricles are larger than expected.

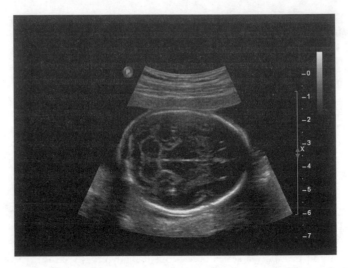

Figure 7.3 A section of the fetal head showing the surrounding skull, the midline between the two brain hemispheres and a posterior brain structure, the cerebellum

Hydrocephaly is often associated with other abnormalities—nearly all fetuses with spina bifida have hydrocephaly too. After birth, babies with hydrocephaly are treated by placing a tube from the enlarged ventricles to the abdomen, to drain off the fluid. Although hydrocephaly can be treated by a drainage procedure before birth, this is rarely done as it does little to reduce the damage from the condition. The outlook for hydrocephaly depends on its cause and severity. If severe hydrocephaly is detected prior to birth there is usually a poor outlook.

Spina bifida results in changes both to the skull shape (called a lemon shaped skull) and the brain (including enlargement of the ventricles and an altered cerebellum—a structure at the back of the brain). A section of the whole length of the spine can be seen in Figure 7.4. It shows each of the vertebrae and the overlying skin. In the presence of spina bifida, there is usually a defect or hole in the skin, and the back wall of the vertebrae in the affected segment of the spine may be absent.

Face and neck

The face is examined to assess the eye sockets, the profile, and the nose. Figure 7.5 shows the eyes and the bridge of the nose. In Figure 7.6

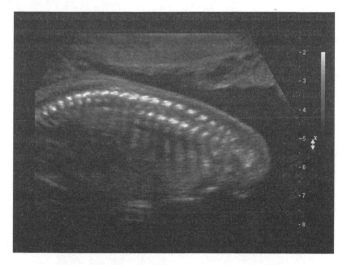

Figure 7.4 A section showing the length of the fetal spine and overlying skin

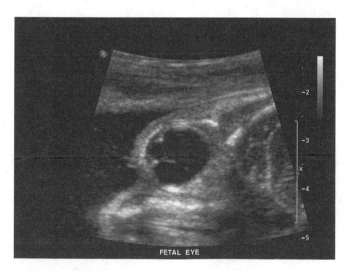

Figure 7.5 Fine detail can be seen of the lens of the eye, the eye socket, and the overlying eyelid

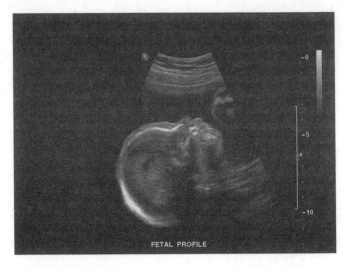

Figure 7.6 Fine 2D profile image

the fetal nose, lips, and chin are visible in profile and the nose can be seen in Figure 7.7 (a). Figure 7.7b shows the line of the upper jaw and the overlying lip.

Facial clefts are the most common abnormality in this area—they occur in about one in 1000 births. Two thirds involve the lip alone, or the lip and the underlying palate. In one third, the palate alone is affected, usually well back in the mouth—but this is unlikely to be diagnosed on ultrasound. With good views of the face, most cleft lips and palates can be detected, but small lesions may be difficult or impossible to see. Nowadays surgical techniques can produce a good cosmetic result, so a good outcome is expected unless there are other problems as well.

Cystic swellings around the neck of the fetus, known as cystic hygromas, occur in approximately one in 200 pregnancies that miscarry, but are uncommon in live-born babies. These are readily diagnosed on ultrasound. The outlook for the baby depends on the degree of swelling of the neck, whether there is swelling elsewhere in the body, and on what has caused the swelling. It is sometimes caused by a chromosomal abnormality, most commonly Turner syndrome (a female with only one X chromosome). Most fetuses with Turner syndrome miscarry, those that do not may have less severe abnormalities. This may include webbing of the neck and an

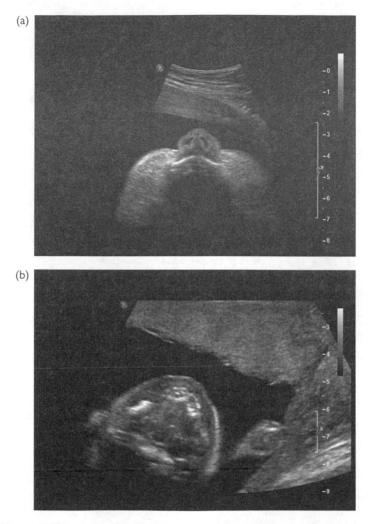

Figure 7.7 Exquisite detail of the nose and the nostrils can also be seen in (a) and the lip and palate in (b) from 18 weeks as long as the views are good

increased likelihood of heart and kidney abnormalities. These children are often of normal intelligence, but there may be some specific learning disabilities. They are small and do not have functioning ovaries—they cannot have children, except by using a donated ovum and in vitro fertilization technology.

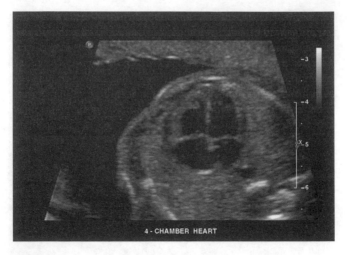

4 - CHAMBER HEART

Figure 7.8 A cross section of the fetal chest shows the four chambers of the heart and allows checking that they are each an appropriate size

Heart and lungs

In the cross-section of the fetal chest shown in Figure 7.8, the four chambers of the heart are visible. If other sections are taken around the heart then the vessels entering and leaving the heart may also be examined.

The heart is examined using both black and white and color images. Red indicates blood flowing up towards the ultrasound transducer and blue is blood flowing away. The technique called Doppler shows flow direction and speed. Doppler increases the chance of picking up holes in the heart and other problems.

There are a large number of structural abnormalities of the heart. They occur in at least one in 125 births and many of them cannot be seen before birth. This is a difficult area of diagnosis and an experienced operator is needed. It is now possible to detect the majority of major structural heart abnormalities at 18 weeks. Advances in cardiac surgery have meant that babies who previously would have died of a heart abnormality may now have surgery after birth. If a heart abnormality is found it is usually recommended that the chromosomes be checked, and the advice of a paediatric heart specialist—a cardiologist—would usually be sought.

Abnormalities of the lungs before birth are rare. The most common problems are cysts on one lung, which is diagnosed when a localized fluid

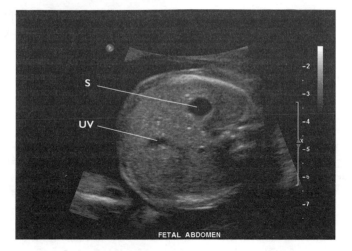

Figure 7.9 A cross section of the fetal abdomen. Notice the abdominal wall and the abdominal contents to be inspected. S = stomach. UV = umbilical vein

collection is seen beside the heart. Even if these cysts are moderately large, they can usually be removed after birth, often with excellent results. Rarely, they need to be drained before birth.

Abdomen and abdominal wall

The section shown in Figure 7.9 is the most important one for checking the growth of the fetus. A deficiency in the skin and muscle of the abdominal wall leads to some of the contents developing outside the abdomen. In omphalocoele—also called exomphalos—there is a membrane covering the bulge, and in gastroschisis there is no membrane. Together, these occur in approximately one in 5000 births. They are usually diagnosed on ultrasound and need no treatment before birth. Most can be closed after birth with good results. Some fetuses with an exomphalos may also have other associated abnormalities—these may be detected with ultrasound or by chromosomal analysis. There are less likely to be other abnormalities with gastroschisis, but bowel damage can occur.

A diaphragmatic hernia is a deficiency in the diaphragm, which causes some of the contents of the abdomen to ride up into the chest. The hernia is most often on the left side of the diaphragm with the stomach sliding up into the chest. Hernias can be surgically treated at birth, but the presence of the abdominal contents in the chest restricts the growth of the lungs.

The adequacy of lung growth is difficult to test before birth, but after birth it may be found that the baby's lung development is inadequate for its survival.

Kidneys

The kidneys are one of the few organs whose function can be assessed before birth. This is done by noting the presence of urine in the bladder and the amount of amniotic fluid. Amniotic fluid is produced when the fetus passes urine. If there is no urine, then there is no amniotic fluid. No amniotic fluid for a prolonged period during pregnancy often results in inadequate lung development which cannot sustain life after birth.

Kidney abnormalities occur in approximately 0.8 per cent of babies. These include the absence of one or both kidneys, cysts, and blockage of the outflow of urine. If both kidneys are absent or totally blocked, the baby usually dies immediately after birth. Fetuses with a blockage of the outflow below the level of the kidneys may occasionally be suitable for treatment by inserting a tube above the level of the blockage to drain urine into the amniotic space (see Chapter 9).

Hydronephrosis is an enlargement of the collecting system of the kidneys. It is usually due to a blockage somewhere in the outflow from the kidneys.

Pyelectasis is the word used to describe a small increase in the amount of fluid in the collecting system of the kidney (see Figure 7.10). Urine from the kidney passes into a collecting chamber in the kidney known as the pelvis (not to be confused with the bony pelvis at the hips). In normal fetuses some urine can often be seen in each pelvis. If the measurement is 4 mm or more it is usually considered to be increased—or pyelectasis. This is not necessarily a problem, but is usually simply a normal variation in size. If the measurement is between 4 and 10 mm, the fetus rarely develops any problem before birth. Some develop what are usually minor problems later in childhood, such as vesico-ureteric reflux. This means that every time the child passes urine, some also flushes back up the tubes towards the kidneys. These children may need treatment with antibiotics and occasionally, if it is severe, surgery. If the condition is recognised early, then long-term damage is unusual.

The proportion of babies with pyelectasis that develop subsequent problems in childhood is low, but the exact number is unclear. It is often worthwhile checking progress with a scan in later pregnancy, and perhaps with investigations after birth, but the outlook is usually excellent. Occasionally, the pelvis of the kidney continues to enlarge during the pregnancy, but it is

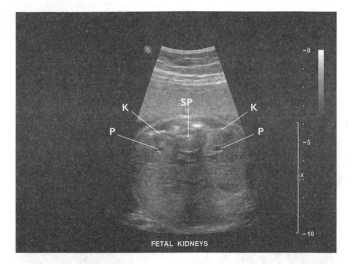

Figure 7.10 A cross section of the fetal abdomen allows the spine (SP) and the two kidneys (K) to be seen. Within each fetal kidney there is a small amount of fluid in the pelvis, the collecting system (P). When the amount of fluid in the pelvis is increased this is called pyelectasis

uncommon for it to enlarge enough to cause kidney damage, so it rarely changes the management of the pregnancy.

It has been suggested that fetuses with an increased amount of fluid in the pelvis of the kidney at around 18 weeks are at higher risk for Down syndrome. But this is a weak connection—see 'markers' page 119.

Limbs

Each limb is inspected during the ultrasound examination. Calcium starts to form in the bones by the end of the third month of pregnancy, and bones stand out as dense white lines. The soft tissues, such as muscles, are seen around the bone. The thigh bone (femur) is usually measured; it is usually easy to measure the length of any long bone.

Dwarfism is diagnosed if the length of the bones in the limbs is well below the normal range. The diagnosis may be made as early as 14–16 weeks, but depending on the cause, it may not be possible to diagnose until 22 weeks or even later. As the pregnancy advances, the limbs of an affected fetus fall increasingly below the normal range. While some babies born with dwarfism lead a normal life, there are a large number who also have abnormalities in other areas of their body. These abnormalities may be so severe with some types of dwarfism that the baby cannot survive after birth.

Bone fractures may occur before birth in conditions such as osteogenesis imperfecta, or brittle bone disease. In this condition the bones break very easily and may be noticeably bent before birth.

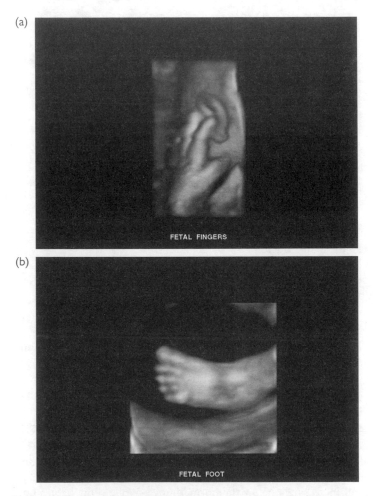

Figure 7.11 Beautiful images of (a) the hand with a finger in the ear, (b) the foot, using 3D ultrasound

Hands and feet

Figure 7.11a shows the hands and fingers. It is usually easy to count the fingers, but this depends on the position of the hand. Sometimes, extra or missing fingers may be difficult to detect. Abnormalities in the shape of the hand or the position of the fingers are occasionally seen.

The feet are easily seen on ultrasound (see Figure 7.11b) and can be checked to ensure that each foot is at the appropriate angle to the lower part of the leg. A severe case of clubfoot can be seen before birth as the foot is turned on the lower leg.

What are markers—or 'soft signs'— of abnormalities?

Markers are changes in the appearance of the physical structure of a fetus that cause no harm in themselves, but are *sometimes* a sign of a more serious condition. The greatest effort has been in detecting markers of chromosome abnormality, particularly Down syndrome. Because Down syndrome is unreliably picked from abnormalities at 18–20 weeks, researchers have focussed on other changes that might give a hint of a fetus having Down syndrome. However, markers are unreliable, they are often seen in fetuses without Down syndrome and Down syndrome fetuses often have no markers.

Most fetuses with Down syndrome have no major structural abnormalities. After birth they have some subtle facial differences, but these cannot be detected with a scan. Some have heart abnormalities or a blockage in the upper part of the intestines, which may be identified on ultrasound. Usually, when an abnormality is detected with ultrasound, it is suggested that the chromosomes be tested to exclude the presence of Down syndrome and other chromosomal abnormalities.

The best marker of Down syndrome is nuchal oedema—swelling in the soft tissues at the back of the neck. Nuchal oedema is a good sign of Down syndrome at 11–14 weeks because the fluid tends to absorb after 14 weeks, but at 18–22 weeks it is still a useful sign (see nuchal translucency scanning, Chapter 5, page 56).

Many other signs of Down syndrome have been reported. They include long bones that are slightly shorter than expected, a bright spot in the middle of one of the pumping chambers of the heart muscle (called echogenic focus), a bright looking fetal bowel (called echogenic bowel), and increased fluid within the collecting system of the kidneys (called pyelectasis).

Nothing that can be seen on an ultrasound examination will tell you for certain if your fetus does have Down syndrome. These signs merely create a suspicion. To confirm or deny this you will need to have either a CVS test or an amniocentesis. Most fetuses with a marker or markers of Down syndrome will be born normal, but the chance of Down syndrome is higher. The more markers present, the higher the risk.

Choroid plexus cysts—markers of trisomy 18

These are small pockets of fluid that become trapped within a collection of tiny blood vessels, called the choroid plexus, in the brain. They are seen in at least 1 in 100 fetuses scanned at 18–22 weeks. These cysts do not cause brain damage, cerebral palsy, or intellectual impairment because they are not present in the brain substance itself. They do not continue to grow during the pregnancy, and usually disappear by around 24 weeks.

The main reason to take notice of choroid plexus cysts is because they are a marker of trisomy 18. That is, they can be a sign that there is an extra chromosome 18—an abnormality known as trisomy 18 or Edward syndrome. Fetuses with trisomy 18 usually die during pregnancy or shortly after birth. Most have other abnormalities, particularly of the heart and limbs. When a choroid plexus cyst is detected, a scan should be carried out by a skilled and experienced operator, using state-of-the-art equipment. If no other abnormality is found, the cyst is usually insignificant.

The chance of trisomy 18 being present when a choroid plexus cyst is seen is linked to the age of the pregnant woman, but is a relatively small risk. For example, the risk of Down syndrome being carried by a pregnant woman at any specified age is greater than the chance of trisomy 18 when the fetus is shown to have choroid plexus cysts but no other abnormality. Because of the relatively low risk, most pregnant women do not choose to have an amniocentesis for choroid plexus cysts alone. Having these cysts does not mean your fetus has an abnormality, but is merely a sign to look for other abnormalities.

It is important that markers of chromosome abnormality are not taken in isolation. The overwhelming likelihood is that even if a marker is found, your baby will be born normal.

What do markers mean?

The presence of a marker should not be greeted with shock or horror. It does not mean there is something the matter; so there may be no need to rush in and do another test. It is a time to pause, and consider the risks of the marker, taking into account other tests that have been done. Different estimates of the risk of a chromosome abnormality with the various markers have been produced, and the figures vary greatly between studies. Any figures can only be an approximation. Some markers, such as those for pyelectasis, increase the risk of Down syndrome very little, if at all. Nuchal thickening of greater than 6 mm does significantly increase the risk of Down syndrome. A best guess figure for the increased risk should be multiplied by the risk of Down syndrome using the age of the pregnant woman and any other tests for Down syndrome that have already been done. Using this strategy, most women with a single marker will remain in the low risk group for Down syndrome. When several markers are found your risk tends to increase much more.

Markers cause great concern largely because people think of them as an abnormality, when they are not. It is frightening to hear that something might be wrong. But it is important not to think of a marker in isolation. If previous testing has given you a low risk figure for Down syndrome, for example, one in 2000, even if a marker is present at 18–22 weeks your chance of Down syndrome remains very low.

Some people believe that markers of Down syndrome at 18–20 weeks have done more harm than good. This is because the markers are such low risk, the studies looking into them have often been poor, and they often cause women a lot of anxiety. Others are great enthusiasts of markers and have established elaborate screening protocols. Love them or hate them, finding a marker puts a doctor in a difficult position—and he or she often feels compelled to discuss it with the pregnant woman.

What are the advantages and disadvantages of an ultrasound examination at 18–22 weeks?

Not everybody wants to have all prenatal tests. A scan at 18–22 weeks looks for a wide range of problems; major, minor, and markers. If you don't want to be told about some minor abnormalities or markers, say this in advance. But be aware that minor abnormalities and markers may be the only sign on ultrasound of more major problems. A turned foot, a clubbed foot, is a relatively minor and usually correctable abnormality. Occasionally a turned foot may be only sign that can be seen on ultrasound of a more serious abnormality. Only by doing further tests, such as an amniocentesis, may a more serious abnormality be detected. On the other hand, in electing not to find out about minor problems, you save yourself the anxiety and worry of a pregnancy in which you know a problem has been found. If you have things you particularly want to be checked, or not to be checked—speak up.

Advantages of ultrasound at 18–22 weeks

An ultrasound at 18–22 weeks is primarily to check the physical structure of your fetus. The advantages of doing so are:

i) Reassurance: Most couples worry a great deal about whether their baby will be normal. A normal scan result gives enormous reassurance, plus the bonding experience of seeing your fetus on the screen.

ii) Choice: If a significant abnormality is found, a couple may decide to have the pregnancy terminated. Couples who decide to continue the pregnancy have the advantage of being forewarned of the abnormality and can research the effect the abnormality is likely to have, and to arrange support for themselves and their child.

iii) Knowledge: Knowing about an abnormality before birth allows medical staff to be forewarned. Some of the abnormalities detected on ultrasound may require urgent treatment at birth if the baby is to have the best chance of healthy survival. This may mean arranging delivery at a hospital where specialists and paediatric facilities are available.

iv) Special arrangements: It is sometimes important to know that an abnormality is present to allow delivery to be brought on early. This helps to minimize the continuing damage from the abnormality before birth. If ultrasound detects blocked kidneys, for example, and the condition deteriorates, the baby may be delivered early and the disease treated.

v) Treatment: Very occasionally specific abnormalities can be treated before birth. Some of these are described in Chapter 9, page 139.

Disadvantages of ultrasound at 18–22 weeks

i) Cost: State of the art equipment is expensive, and it costs money to train people to operate it. The cost of scans and other tests excludes lower income women in some health care systems.

ii) Biological effects of ultrasound: There have been many ultrasound 'scares' over the years. Although experts say the risks of ultrasound are low, the evidence on potential ill-effects is incomplete.

iii) Seeing something that is not there: One of the major skills of people who interpret ultrasound scans is to decide whether something that looks different is different and normal, or different and abnormal. With experience, a doctor can often be confident about whether a difference matters, but sometimes other tests may be needed. 'Markers' show an increased risk of an abnormality, but are not themselves abnormalities.

iv) Missed abnormalities: Ultrasound operators are fallible, and sometimes abnormalities that should be picked up are missed. Ultrasound cannot pick up everything—sometimes a difficult view means that something is missed, or it may simply be too early to see a specific condition. Some very difficult diagnoses could not be expected in an ordinary clinical setting.

What happens if an abnormality is found at 18–22 weeks?

If an abnormality is found, then the treatment options vary with the personal beliefs of the pregnant woman, the severity of the abnormality, and local laws.

Before even considering treatment options, it is important to get full and reliable information about the abnormality that has been found. Don't forget that you decide on the management of your pregnancy.

The internet is a great resource, but some websites are more accurate than others (see Chapter 10 for contacts). Discuss your concerns with experts in your local area. One of the major improvements in the care of pregnant women with fetal abnormalities, has been the development of multidisciplinary groups where women can get advice from experts in different areas of medicine. This group of specialists often includes a geneticist, a neonatal paediatrician and a paediatrician specialising in the particular abnormality that has been detected. If there is no such group in your area, you should still make contact with local experts who specialise in the appropriate area. It can be very useful to speak to a paediatrician who treats babies with the condition that has been detected in your fetus, as you will find out about how the abnormality might affect your baby and any treatments that are available. It is also important to find out the risks of other abnormalities that may *not* be detected before birth.

The prime goal of prenatal diagnosis is to maximise information for pregnant women so that they may make informed choices.

What are the treatment options at 18–22 weeks?

Watching and waiting: You do not need to do anything. Some women with very major fetal abnormalities choose to continue their pregnancy. Others choose to terminate a pregnancy with less severe abnormalities, often because they fear further problems after birth.

Observing and monitoring: When an abnormality has been found, it is often checked several times later on in the pregnancy. This applies to heart abnormalities and conditions such as hydronephrosis (blocked kidneys).

Early delivery: This may be necessary, particularly if a condition is found to be worsening during the monitoring stage.

Delivery in a major specialist centre: There are some abnormalities where early specialist treatment from paediatricians and paediatric intensive care facilities will improve the baby's healthy survival. This applies particularly to some heart abnormalities and to many others when early treatment may be necessary.

Prenatal treatment: There are a number of prenatal treatments now available including key hole surgery (using a fine telescopic instrument, called a fetoscope), and ultrasound guided treatments such as draining fluid filled cavities by inserting a tube, or a shunt. These are discussed in Chapter 9. Although fetal surgery attracts a lot of interest, there are very few conditions in which the outcome can be improved by operating before birth. In addition, fetal surgery can pose very significant risks to the woman herself.

Abortion: Many women choose to have an abortion, particularly when a major abnormality has been diagnosed.

Questions about prenatal tests at 18–22 weeks

Can an 18–22 week ultrasound scan pick all abnormalities?
No. All prenatal tests are designed to detect a specific range of abnormalities. Ultrasound at this stage of pregnancy is an excellent way of detecting many, but not all, of the major physical abnormalities. There are many problems that it cannot detect. For example, it is of limited value in detecting how organs function. It cannot assess brain functions and detect intellectual impairment or cerebral palsy. On the positive side, it is an excellent screening test for many major physical abnormalities.

Is there always a problem if a marker of Down syndrome is identified?
No. Markers are not abnormalities. They merely identify an increased risk, and often a small increase in the risk, of abnormality. The vast majority of babies born after a marker has been found are healthy and normal.

Will I be able to tell the sex on the scan?
No. It is rare for couples to be able to identify the sex unless they are experienced looking at ultrasound scans. Very occasionally couples can identify the male penis but it is difficult to differentiate from other structures, such as the cord.

Is 3D ultrasound better than 2D?
No. Most medical diagnoses are made with 2D ultrasound. 3D is increasingly being used but still has a relatively small place in making an initial diagnosis.

Is it OK to go for a 'shopping mall' 3D or 4D ultrasound scan, so I can get some good pictures?
Medical opinion varies on this issue. In general, how you spend your money is your decision but there are a number of potential problems with having an ultrasound scan for non-medical purposes, and many doctors have reservations. An abnormality may be missed. An abnormality may be seen that may then present some management problems. A big factor is that these are expensive and potentially reduce a couples capacity to pay for useful medical interventions. Most doctors believe that it is better to enjoy the ultrasound scan that it is carried out for a serious medical purpose.

Could other technologies replace ultrasound?
The magnificent images produced by magnetic resonance imaging (MRI) means that MRI has a role after an abnormality has been found on ultrasound. It can be used to confirm ultrasound diagnoses and it provides improved tissue detail and assessment of function. But MRI scans are relatively expensive and they cannot currently produce moving, or real time, images, so its role remains limited.

What about ultrasound in the future?

It is not possible to look into a crystal ball to see where ultrasound will be in 10 or 20 years. However, the magnificent images that can be produced with ultrasound, plus its safety record, combine to ensure that ultrasound will remain the pivotal technology in prenatal testing well into the future.

Much of the current research and excitement about 3D and 4D ultrasound among the medical profession is its potential for the future. It may be useful for 'deskilling' the job of an ultrasound operator, because a less experienced operator in a geographically isolated area could send a volume of information to a central site for an expert to examine.

There is no doubt that an increasing role for 3D ultrasound will be found with time. In 10 years 3D and 4D ultrasound will have a much bigger role in diagnosing a problem. Continued refinements in computer processing techniques will result in ongoing improvements in imaging. This will allow increasing numbers of diagnoses to be made earlier and earlier in pregnancy.

8 Prenatal testing: 23 weeks until delivery

Prenatal testing for abnormalities is carried out much less often from 23 weeks of pregnancy until delivery. At this stage, testing is aimed at identifying problems with your baby's growth or following up a problem that was identified earlier on. The two main forms of prenatal testing that are done late in pregnancy are checking your baby's heart rate, and an ultrasound examination. Occasionally amniocentesis and magnetic resonance imaging are performed.

It is not usual to perform prenatal tests late in pregnancy unless there is a problem with the mother or the baby that puts the pregnancy at risk. This assumes that the mother has received appropriate prenatal care up to this point and that she is continuing to see her doctor or midwife in late pregnancy for regular examinations.

What does the baby look like at 23 weeks?

The baby is completely developed at this stage. At 23 weeks the average baby weighs a little over 454 gms (1 pound) and by 40 weeks it will have grown to an average of about 3150 gms (7½ pounds). At 23 weeks babies can begin to survive outside the uterus, but they are very fragile and will need a lot of help with breathing. They may experience many other medical problems because they are so premature. Babies born at 22 weeks or less rarely survive because their lungs are not developed enough to exchange air. Over 70 per cent of babies born at 24 weeks will survive if they are born at a hospital with an advanced neonatal nursing facilities and care. Many hospitals or centers will have calculated their own survival rates.

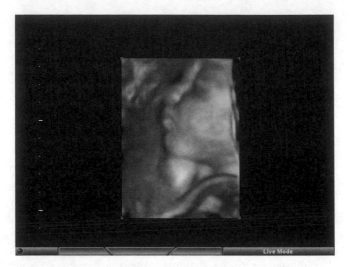

Figure 8.1 3D image of the fetus late in pregnancy

Why would I be offered prenatal tests at this stage of pregnancy?

If the mother has health problems

Certain medical condition put your pregnancy at higher risk, and doctors may want to check your baby's growth and well-being. These conditions include high blood pressure, diabetes, kidney, cardiac, collagen, and vascular diseases. Mothers who smoke, drink alcohol, and use either prescription or recreational drugs are also in this high risk category. Depending on the findings, the mother may be hospitalized, given medical treatment or advised to consider an early delivery.

If there are problems with the pregnancy

Complications that put you or your baby at a higher risk include premature labor, pre-eclampsia, premature rupture of the membranes, a baby that feels too large or too small, or bleeding late in pregnancy. It is important to check the baby's growth and well-being in such pregnancies.

If you have a multiple pregnancy or are overdue

Women with twins or multiple babies might also be offered late testing. If it hasn't been done already, it is important to find out if twins share one placenta. Those that do, are at a higher risk than those that do not. Even if there have been no complications in a particular pregnancy, it is possible that you will be offered tests if you are overdue.

What tests can be done at 23 weeks, or more, of pregnancy?

The two most common tests are fetal heart rate testing and an ultrasound examination.

Fetal heart rate monitoring is called the 'non-stress test'. During this test, a monitor is placed on your abdomen and the pattern of your baby's heart rate is recorded and interpreted, while you record your baby's movements. The doctor or midwife looks if the baby's heart rate increases when it is moving. If this happens the test is called 'reactive' and it indicates a healthy baby. A repeat examination is usually done one week later, sometimes sooner.

An ultrasound examination, similar to the scan done earlier in pregnancy, can be done at any time, including just before or even during labor. It aims to check the following:

How your baby is growing: Your baby's weight is estimated to see if it is too big or too small. This estimate can be inaccurate, as the exact weight of the baby cannot be known before birth. It may need to be checked again after two weeks.

How much amniotic fluid is present and the position of the placenta: If there is too little amniotic fluid, this may be a sign that the placenta is not supplying the baby with blood. Examination of the placenta may show that it is not in a good location. It may be in front of the baby (placenta previa) or it may have a blood clot behind it (abruptio placenta). The way the baby is facing can also be seen on ultrasound. This information is especially important in twin pregnancies, and can help the obstetrician determine how the baby (or babies) should be delivered.

How your baby is breathing and moving: Doctors will look at how your baby is breathing and moving inside the uterus to assess how healthy it is. This is called a 'biophysical profile'.

The blood flow: Doppler ultrasound can check the blood flow in the mother's or the baby's blood vessels, or in the umbilical cord.

If there is an abnormality, such as fluid in the kidney, further ultrasound scans may be scheduled at fixed intervals to follow the problem and to make sure it does not get worse. Less common tests you might be offered at this stage of pregnancy are magnetic resonance imaging and amniocentesis (see pages 130–131).

Can you see the baby better on ultrasound at 23 weeks or more?

You might think it is easier to see the baby late in pregnancy and you might expect better pictures than before. But these late ultrasound images are often disappointing, because there is less room for the baby and less amniotic fluid in proportion to its size. You might not be able to see your baby's face at all if it is in the wrong position, or you might be lucky and get a good view. What you see depends on technical factors, including the baby's position and the amount of amniotic fluid.

How accurate is ultrasound at detecting abnormalities at this stage?

Abnormalities can still be detected at this stage of pregnancy, although this later examination does not usually focus as much on the baby's anatomy. If an earlier ultrasound has not been done, a careful evaluation of the baby's anatomy should be performed at this stage.

Some abnormalities may not be seen until late in pregnancy. An example of this includes microcephaly—a head that is smaller than it should be. There are also some kidney or bowel problems and some tumours that can show up later on, even if earlier examinations were done correctly and showed normal results. These conditions are not normally looked for in earlier ultrasound examinations but they may be detected during an ultrasound that is performed later and for other reasons.

Can amniocentesis be done late in pregnancy?

Amniocentesis can be used late in pregnancy, to determine if the baby's lungs are mature. This is done by looking for certain substances in the amniotic fluid that are produced by mature fetal lungs, such as lecithin and phosphatidylglycerol. Usually this is not necessary, unless there is a medical or obstetrical complication. For example if there was a previous vertical scar on the uterus and the doctor wanted to deliver the baby early, but only if the baby's lungs were mature. In other situations, such as premature labor or premature rupture of the membranes, some doctors will perform an amniocentesis to look for signs of infection as well as fetal lung maturity, to help them decide what to do.

It is uncommon to perform an amniocentesis late in pregnancy to check if the baby's chromosomes are normal, because it may be too late to consider ending the pregnancy. It could still done, however, to assist the doctor and the couple in decision making (see Chapter 9). An amniocentesis at this stage can tell you if your baby has a serious problem for which nothing can be done. The rapid form of chromosome testing called fluorescent in-situ hybridization or FISH (see Chapters 5 and 6) may be used to detect the more common abnormalities, in situations where the results are needed faster than usual.

When would magnetic resonance imaging be done?

In rare cases, magnetic resonance imaging (MRI) can be of value in accurately diagnosing an abnormality such as a brain disorder. This can help the doctor to advise the couple regarding likely outcomes and management options. Until recently, MRI had very limited usefulness because the baby's movements meant poor quality images. Improvements in technology mean that good images can now be obtained. However, ultrasound is just as good as MRI in almost all circumstances. MRI costs much more and is sometimes more uncomfortable because the examination is often done in a confining space. Occasionally, the information obtained by ultrasound in cases of a brain abnormality, a hole in the baby's diaphragm, or a placenta that is growing into the uterus, can be enhanced by the additional information gained from MRI.

9 Decisions after prenatal testing

If an abnormality is detected, you have several options for your pregnancy. Before you make any decisions, you will need the best information possible, including professional advice. Your most important choice will be whether to continue with or end your pregnancy. If you decide to continue your pregnancy you will face other options. You may also be concerned about becoming pregnant again.

When a problem with an unborn baby is detected, it is usually unexpected. About 3 per cent of all pregnancies will be affected by some fetal abnormality. This is roughly the equivalent of correctly guessing the right number before a spin of a roulette wheel. Even if you had counseling before the test, an abnormal result still comes as a big shock. Almost always, there is nothing that you did or did not do to cause the problem. All women are at risk when they become pregnant. It may be some time later, after you have experienced disbelief, shock, and sometimes unwarranted guilt, when you can start to think about what to do. Before you make any decisions you need to get the best information.

Megan and her husband, Joseph, had every expectation that their baby would be normal. This was their first pregnancy. They were a young and healthy working couple and had no family history of any problem. The ultrasound showed that their baby had excess fluid in its brain or hydrocephalus. In their case, this type of hydrocephalus was associated with a high risk of severe intellectual handicap. Their first reaction was anger at the doctor who broke the news to them. Subsequently, they asked for another opinion because they could not believe that their baby was not going to be normal. During this process, Megan wondered if there was anything that she had done, or did not do, that caused this problem.

Where can I get the best information?

The best place to start is to talk to your doctor, or midwife. Make sure that you understand what the actual problem is. Sometimes the exact nature of the problem and the outcome for your baby is uncertain. A repeat ultrasound examination may be recommended to gather more information. It can be very useful to discuss your situation with an obstetrician (a doctor specializing in pregnancy and birth), a paediatrician (child health specialist), or a genetic counselor. Charities or voluntary organizations, such as support and self-help groups for specific conditions, are another valuable source of information. They can provide information, support, and put you in touch with other parents of children with the same problem. See Contacts, page 153.

Many people use the internet for health information, but it can be difficult to determine the quality of that information. Material from professional or governmental organizations is a reliable source, see Chapter 10, page 153. Specialists working at academic medical centers and universities who concentrate or do research in a particular area can also be a useful resource.

Megan and Joseph (see previous page), sought a consultation with a specialist at a medical center in their city who was well known for his expertise in diagnosing problems with the fetal brain. He confirmed their worst fear and referred them to a pediatric neurosurgeon. The neurosurgeon informed them of the range of outcomes that might occur as well as the procedures that would be needed after the baby was born to relieve the pressure on its brain. He told them about other children that he had treated with this condition and suggested they contact a support group to ask these parents what their experiences had been.

Making a decision if an abnormality is found

After getting all the information you need, and making sure you fully understand your options, you, and your partner if you have one, will have to make a decision about how to proceed. Other members of your family such as parents and siblings, along with close friends, may be able to help you as well. But too much well-meaning and contradicting advice can be confusing. We recommend that you limit the friends and family who you talk to. Depending upon your religious beliefs, you may also choose to talk to a member of your clergy. Some doctors, or midwives, may be able to give counseling as well as medical information. You can decide who to talk to and whether you should follow their advice.

Megan and Joseph were devout Catholics and they decided to discuss the problem with their parish priest as well as their own parents, who had been very excited about the birth of their first grandchild. Their doctor reassured them that any decision that they made would be the right decision for them.

What are my options?

Your choices are to some extent dependent on what stage your pregnancy is at when the problem is found, how clear or certain the diagnosis is, and the abortion laws in your area. Your main options are to end your pregnancy, by having an abortion (see pages 135–138) or to continue with your pregnancy. In rare cases, treatment can be given before birth (see pages 138–143).

Whatever abnormality is found—major or minor—you do not have to do anything. You might simply decide to let nature take its course. Some abnormalities turn out not to be as severe as they were predicted. Others can be prepared for; you could decide to get information from experts, support groups, and other parents with affected babies. For some conditions, such as a cleft lip (harelip), it can be useful to learn the special feeding techniques before your baby is born. Sadly, some conditions are so severe that the parents make the decision to allow the baby to die while still inside the uterus or shortly after birth.

Rachel and Steven had a fetus that was diagnosed with anencephaly, which is the failure of the brain to completely develop. They decided not to have an abortion but they knew that there was nothing that could be done for the baby once it was born. When Rachel went into labor, she was not monitored and when the baby was born alive, the child was given only comfort care. It died in a few days and Rachel and Steven arranged for a burial according to their religious tradition.

If you continue with your pregnancy, your baby may be closely observed and arrangements made for delivering it in a specialist center or hospital with experts on hand. Sometimes, delivery by Cesarean section, or, less commonly, early delivery may give the baby the best chance of healthy survival.

Many women choose to have an abortion (see page 135), particularly when a major abnormality has been diagnosed. For most women, choosing to end their pregnancy by having an abortion is one of the most agonizing and difficult decisions that they will ever face. There are some couples for whom abortion is not an option, either because of their religious or personal beliefs, but who do not think that they can raise the child themselves.

In such cases, adoption can also be an option. Fortunately, some individuals and groups feel that they are able to raise children with special needs and are dedicated to providing homes for children with even severe disabilities.

Should I try again?

When a baby dies either before or after birth, or if a child is born with a problem, couples often doubt their ability to have a normal child. Find out as much as you can about your pregnancy, including an autopsy if possible, so that you can get the best information for going forward. There are some problems that are unlikely to happen again, and that will make no difference to future pregnancies. There are others with a genetic link that may put future pregnancies at an increased risk. There are some conditions for which prevention may be possible, such as treatment with folic acid to prevent spinal defects, or controlling your diabetes to prevent heart and other defects. That is why it is important to seek counseling before you try to become pregnant again.

What will happen if I choose to have an abortion?

Abortion is a medically safe procedure when performed by a competent doctor. During the first 3 months, there are two basic options; a medical abortion that can only be done very early (up to 7 weeks), or a surgical abortion that is usually done after 7 weeks and up to 12 to 13 weeks of pregnancy. You should discuss with your doctor what method is suggested, where and by whom it will be done, and what you can expect to happen before, during, and after the procedure.

Medical abortion before 7 weeks

In a medical abortion drugs called Mifepristone or Methotrexate, alone or in combination with another drug, Misoprostol, are used to end a pregnancy. These drugs can only be taken if you are less than about 7 weeks pregnant—so they cannot be used by most women who wish to terminate a pregnancy. The advantage of a medical abortion is that it does not involve surgery or anesthesia—the medication can be taken in the privacy of your own home. This method is only 90–95 per cent effective so it is important to get medical follow-up.

Mifepristone is taken orally. It is still not available in Australia. It blocks the action of progesterone and causes the lining of the uterus to become thinner so that the egg will detach. It also causes the opening of the womb—called the cervix—to dilate while increasing the production of hormones that cause contractions. Methotrexate is given by injection 1 week before the other drugs. It causes the embryo and the supporting tissues to stop growing. Misoprostol and mifepristone are usually given orally at the same time. These help to stimulate contractions to empty the uterus. In the UK, Mifepristone is used and then Misoprostal 48 hours later; Methotrexate is not used at all.

Most abnormalities are discovered too late for a medical abortion. This procedure is not as effective as a surgical abortion, and you need to visit your doctor or medical center at least two or three times. Like all medical procedures, there can be complications. These include heavy or prolonged vaginal bleeding, infection, and incomplete removal of the embryo. In addition, many women find actually seeing the embryo upsetting or unpleasant. A surgical abortion may sometimes need to be done afterwards to complete the procedure or to stop the heavy bleeding.

You should not have a medical abortion if you have any clotting problems or are taking anti-clotting medication, or if you have heart, lung, or kidney disease. You should not have a medical abortion if you cannot return to the doctor or are unwilling to accept the chance that you may need a surgical abortion afterwards if the medication does not work.

Surgical abortion before 13 weeks

In a surgical abortion, thin tapered metal rods or dilators are inserted into the cervix to open it. A tube is then placed inside the uterus with suction attached. The contents of the uterus are then sucked out. This procedure requires some type of anaesthetic and you can choose a local or a general. If done correctly, a surgical abortion is more than 99 per cent effective, and it is completed quickly. The vaginal bleeding afterwards is usually shorter and lighter than after a medical abortion.

There is some risk with any surgical procedure. In less than 1 in 100 cases, the abortion is incomplete and may need to be done again. As with a medical abortion, there is the risk of heavy bleeding and infection. The chance of an injury to the uterus or other organs is less than 5 in 1000. These injuries are usually minor, although they may require surgery, including a hysterectomy in very rare cases.

Abortion at 13–24 weeks

At the end of the third month of pregnancy, when the baby and the uterus are larger, abortion is more difficult and more risky. In addition, there may be local laws that put limits on how late an abortion may be performed.

Dilatation and evacuation (D&E)

One of the most common procedures used at this time of pregnancy is a dilatation and evacuation, known as a D&E. This procedure is similar to a dilatation and curettage, or D&C. The cervix, which may need to be prepared the day before by softening it using drugs, is gradually opened with thin metal dilators. Special tools are used to remove the fetus, often in parts. The fetal nervous system is not very developed at this point and it is unlikely that it can feel pain. You will need some kind of anesthesia for this procedure; you can choose a local or general anaesthetic. Complications such as rupture of the uterus, excessive bleeding, perforation of the uterus or infection can occur, but these are rare when the procedure is done by an experienced person in a hospital or specially equipped clinic.

Induction of labor

Another option for abortion after 13 weeks is to induce labor. This is usually done with synthetic hormones that are placed in the uterus with a needle, or inserted as a suppository (pessary) into the vagina. This type of procedure takes much longer as the fetus has to be delivered, and the woman usually experiences labor pains. Sometimes, the fetus may be born alive and will be allowed to die. In other cases, doctors will use ultrasound guidance to inject potassium chloride into the fetus so that it will not be born alive.

What happens if I am carrying twins or have a multiple pregnancy?

In a multiple pregnancy where only one of the fetuses has been diagnosed with a problem, it may be possible to abort that fetus without affecting the other(s). This is called selective termination and is done by injecting potassium into the heart of the affected fetus. There is a small risk that this procedure can adversely affect the normal fetus, by introducing infection or by causing the mother to go into premature labor. In the rare cases where this procedure is considered, you should talk to an expert who is familiar with it.

Some women choose to reduce the number of fetuses that they are carrying even if no problem has been found with any of them. This can happen after some infertility treatment when there are three or more fetuses. If you are considering this procedure, you need up to date information on what outcome can be expected if you have a reduction of pregnancy, or if you leave things as they are.

What can I expect after an abortion?

Medical consequences

You may worry about your ability to become pregnant again. For most women, a previous abortion will have no effect on your ability to become pregnant again, or to carry another pregnancy to 40 weeks. In rare cases, depending on the procedure that you had, the neck of your cervix may become weak and may need to be checked more often during a subsequent pregnancy. If there is a complication during the abortion, which happens rarely, your ability to become pregnant in the future, or your ability to carry a pregnancy to 40 weeks and deliver normally may be affected. While abortion does have some risks, an early abortion has been shown to be safer overall than continuing a pregnancy and delivering at 40 weeks.

Psychological consequences

Almost all women have some emotional response to an abortion. Counseling before and afterwards is recommended—ask your doctor to recommend somebody. Because views on abortion vary depending on background and religious and ethical beliefs, women who have an abortion are affected differently. Reactions can be severe, unpredictable, and unexpected. In a more advanced pregnancy, you are likely to feel some bonding, especially if you have seen your baby on an ultrasound scan or if you have felt it move.

Your decision to have an abortion should be carefully thought out beforehand and you should be prepared for some time of mourning afterwards. There is often grief for the baby that is lost and for the child that you have started to anticipate. You should decide whether you want to see the baby when it is delivered, if this is possible. This may be an especially difficult time for you if either your pregnancy or the abortion has been kept secret from family members and friends. Women who choose to have an abortion often lack the social support that is given if a baby dies in pregnancy through natural causes.

Are any treatments available before my baby is born?

There are no prenatal treatments for most abnormalities, but in rare cases, treatment is available. This includes giving drugs, intrauterine blood transfusion, draining fluid filled cavities and surgery on your unborn baby. See opposite for details.

Drug treatment

In rare cases, drugs are used to help fetal heart rate abnormalities, especially a very fast fetal heart rate. Fetal infections such as toxoplasmosis may be treated with antibiotics.

Fetal blood transfusion and stem cell transplantation

Some blood disorders can be treated prenatally. These include when the baby's blood type is not compatible with its mother's or when the baby has a risk of bleeding because there are too few platelets. The fetus is treated by placing a needle into the umbilical cord—guided by ultrasound—testing the blood and then giving blood or blood products to the baby. Fetal blood transfusions were the first fetal treatments ever carried out. It has now become a very successful and accepted treatment, although it is rarely needed.

Congenital immunodeficiencies, such as severe combined immunodeficiency disease can result in severe infection after birth and early death. Doctors have attempted to transplant stem cells into the fetal circulation in the same way as a blood transfusion. Gene therapy has also been considered to correct certain problems before the baby is born. Whether these procedures are successful depends on the specific condition that the fetus has, and the current state of knowledge about how best to treat it. Doctors are learning more about stem cells and gene therapy everyday.

Draining fluid-filled cavities

If there is fluid around the baby's lungs, drainage may be helpful. A needle is inserted and the fluid is drawn out of the chest cavity. Drainage of other fluid filled collections, such as fluid-filled cysts in other parts of the body may be recommended in extremely rare cases.

Fetal surgery

Most abnormalities cannot be corrected during your pregnancy. There are a few life-threatening conditions for which fetal surgery has been tried and has been successful, although these procedures are often very risky. Surgery may be tried for conditions that are diagnosed when the fetus is too immature to be delivered; and when waiting until it is more developed may be too late to fix the problem. In these cases the experts hope that correcting the problem as early as possible will prevent further complications as the pregnancy progresses.

Most of these procedures are considered experimental and should only be attempted in the few specialized hospitals or centers where pediatric surgeons, maternal–fetal medicine experts and other specialists are working as part of a team to develop and perfect them. Since these conditions are rare, only a few centers have enough real experience in performing them.

There is much that modern obstetrics can do to improve the outcome for a baby with abnormalities, without resorting to invasive fetal surgery.

How is fetal surgery done?

Before having this treatment, you should be given information and counseling about what to expect. There are two main types of procedures in fetal surgery:

Open fetal surgery—the uterus is opened, the fetus is partially removed and surgery is done to correct the problem. Afterward the fetus is replaced inside the uterus, and drugs are given to try and prevent the pregnant woman from going into labor.

Fetoscopic surgery—a fiberoptic telescope with special instruments is inserted through a very small hole in the woman's skin and uterus. This type of surgery is less traumatic and has a smaller risk of causing premature labor.

What are the risks of fetal surgery?

All these procedures have serious potential risks. The major risks are premature labor that cannot be stopped, causing the baby to be delivered too early, or problems for the pregnant woman. These could include bleeding or infection, plus complications from the drugs or anesthesia that is used. If there is a scar in the uterus from an open fetal surgical procedure, there may be an increased risk of the uterus rupturing during a subsequent pregnancy.

What types of problems might be helped with fetal surgery?

When the passage of urine is blocked

After about 14 weeks of pregnancy, the fetus's urine makes up the amniotic fluid that surrounds it. If there is a blockage to the flow of urine, for example, caused by an undeveloped urethra (the tube that drains the bladder), then the fetal kidneys may be damaged by a back-up of urine and its lungs underdeveloped because of the insufficient amniotic fluid. Both the kidney damage and the small lungs may be life-threatening to the fetus.

One of the first procedures performed prenatally was to relieve a blockage in an unborn baby's urethra. This involves placing a tube with a valve, called a shunt, into the bladder, with the help of ultrasound. This temporary shunt can drain the fluid into the amniotic cavity until the baby is delivered, when the problem can be surgically repaired. While the blockage of urine can be relieved, these babies are often left with many medical problems. Recently, removal of the urethral blockage has been attempted through fetoscopy.

Almost always, blockages of the fetal urinary system are mild or only on one side. Surgery is not necessary in these cases, and it is safer to observe the fetus closely with ultrasound, and to carefully examine the child when it is born. A shunt is usually only considered when there is total blockage to urine flow.

When the abdomen has not developed as it should

There are a few conditions affecting the baby's abdomen that may be treated by fetal surgery. Congenital diaphragmatic hernia occurs when the diaphragm, the thin muscle that separates the chest from the abdomen, is partially absent. The intestines may grow into the chest cavity and prevent the lungs from developing properly. The lungs may be too small for the baby to survive after birth. In such cases, pediatric surgeons have attempted to remove the fetus and repair the hole in the diaphragm so the lungs can develop normally. At times, the baby's windpipe can be compressed during the procedure so that the lungs may expand.

Most other abdominal abnormalities are treated after the baby is born. These include gastroschisis, where the contents of the bowel are outside of the abdominal wall, or omphalocoele, where there is a hernia or a protusion of a part of the abdominal wall containing the bowel, the liver, or both. Knowing that these problems are there can help the doctors and the parents to be prepared once the baby is born. Such preparations might include consultations with the pediatric surgeons and decisions to deliver in a hospital where they have experience in taking care of a baby with these problems.

When the fetus has a tumor

There are a few tumors for which fetal surgery has been attempted. These include sacrococcygeal teratoma, which is a large tumor at the base of the baby's spine. If the tumor is very large, the baby's heart may fail because the tumor needs so much of the blood supply. Open fetal surgery has been done to cut off the tumor and replace the fetus in the uterus so that it can develop normally. In other cases, doctors have attempted to cut off the tumor's blood supply with a laser using an endoscope—a thin telescope-like device that allows doctors to see inside the uterus.

If there is a large tumour on the baby's neck, it may obstruct the airway causing amniotic fluid that would otherwise have been swallowed, to accumulate. The excessive amniotic fluid places the pregnant woman at risk of going into labor early. A large tumor makes resuscitation difficult when the baby is born and it cannot breathe. In some cases, it may be appropriate to perform fetal surgery to open the airway and to remove all or part of the tumour. The fetus can then be replaced in the uterus and can continue to grow.

When the spine has not developed as it should

Open fetal surgery has been tried for spina bifida, in the hope that fixing the defect in the spine earlier in pregnancy will lessen the damage and that the baby will have better use of their legs. In addition, it is hoped that the surgery will prevent excess fluid from accumulating in the brain—which often happens when a fetus has a defect in the spine. Pediatric surgeons are now collecting data to find out if correcting this problem while the fetus is still inside the uterus makes a difference in the long term for these children.

Christine and Robert were told that their baby had spina bifida. After counseling, they decided to enroll in a clinical trial where they and their baby were randomly put into one of two groups. One group would be given fetal surgery, while the other would not have any surgery. While they were not sure that their own baby would benefit, they wanted to help advance medical knowledge, so that couples in the future would know if the surgery is truly beneficial.

Twin-to-twin transfusion

When there are identical twins, they may share the same blood supply. Sometimes one fetus can get too much blood and the other too little. If this is happening, doctors can sever the vessels that connect the twins, using an endoscope. This has been successful in many cases. Another option which can help both twins, is to remove the excessive amniotic fluid of one twin, often on several occasions, to try to equalize the pressure in both sacs. Occasionally, if one fetus is very sick, tying off its umbilical cord can save its co-twin.

How often does fetal surgery work?

These procedures are mostly experimental—there are ongoing randomized trials and evaluation is being done. It is a mistake to think of fetal surgery as an established treatment before it has been proven to be of benefit.

It is important to make sure that the diagnosis of abnormality is correct if you are considering fetal surgery. Your doctor will also check, as far as possible, that the fetus does not have any other abnormalities such as heart problems or chromosomal problems that may also affect your pregnancy or your decision. If you are offered fetal surgery, you need to get proper information and counseling. In particular, you should be aware of the risks, such as premature delivery, which can cause problems after your baby is born.

10   Glossary of Terms

Abnormality or anomaly: A physical or chromosome defect found in a fetus.

Abortion: There are two types: an induced abortion (also called a termination of pregnancy or therapeutic abortion) is the deliberate interruption of pregnancy by either surgical or medical means. A spontaneous abortion (also known as a miscarriage) is the natural loss of a pregnancy.

AFP: (see **alpha-fetoprotein**)

Alpha-fetoprotein (AFP): This is a protein in the fetal circulation, some of which passes into the amniotic fluid, and an even smaller amount into the blood stream of the pregnant woman (maternal serum AFP). AFP levels rise in the maternal blood and amniotic fluid of fetuses with NTDs. The level tends to be low in the blood of the pregnant woman when the fetus has Down syndrome, and is one of the substances tested in screening for Down syndrome.

Amniocentesis: A test in which a fine needle is passed through the skin of the pregnant woman into the amniotic sac and a sample of amniotic fluid removed. It is usually done at 15–17 weeks. An early amniocentesis may be done at 12–14 weeks.

Anencephaly: A condition in which the bones of the skull do not form. This usually results in the baby's death shortly after birth because of the severe brain destruction.

Autosome: Any chromosome, except one of the sex chromosomes. There are normally 46 chromosomes of which 2, the X and Y, are the sex chromosomes. The remaining 22 pairs are autosomes.

Blighted ovum: An anembryonic pregnancy, or a pregnancy when the amniotic sac and its surrounding placenta (trophoblast) can be identified, but the fetus cannot be seen. It is common for the fetus to die before 6 weeks after the last period, when it is too small to be seen using ultrasound or at pathology examination. If the fetus dies after 6 weeks it can usually be seen at an ultrasound examination and may be called a missed abortion. This term is inaccurate as it has not been missed by anybody—it usually takes some time for the death of a fetus to be recognized.

Chorionic villus sampling (CVS): A test which involves taking a small piece of placenta. It can be carried out either through the pregnant woman's abdomen (transabdominal CVS) or through the cervix (transcervical CVS). Before 10 weeks, the placenta is called the chorion. Under a microscope it is seen to be full of small tissue projections called villi.

Chorionicity: The number of separate functioning placentas in a twin pregnancy. Most identical twins are monochorionic and their circulations mix. Non-identical twins are always dichorionic. Even if their placentas are joined, there is no communication between the two circulations.

Choroid plexus cyst: A localized collection of fluid within the choroid plexus, a collection of blood vessels, next to the fluid filled chambers of the brain (the ventricles).

Chromosomes: Thread-like structures which occur in pairs in every cell of the body. There are normally 46 chromosomes. Each chromosome carries many genes, which are responsible for a person's inherited characteristics.

Chromosome abnormality: An error in the structure or number of chromosomes.

Cleft lip and palate: A split or defect in the upper lip and palate. A cleft lip may extend to the nose. Where there is a cleft lip it commonly extends back as a gap in the palate.

Club foot: When the foot is turned out of position.

Conception: The start of a pregnancy, that is, the fertilization of a woman's egg by a man's sperm.

Congenital: Present at birth. A congenital abnormality, such as congenital heart disease, is present in a baby at birth. Prenatal testing in the first half of pregnancy enables the detection of many, but not all, congenital abnormalities.

Corpus luteum: The ovulation cyst. After the release of the egg from the ovarian follicle, a cyst forms that is usually 2–5 cm in diameter, this is the corpus luteum. It produces hormones that help to maintain the early pregnancy. It is visible for the first few months with ultrasound.

Crown–rump length: The measurement from the top of the fetal head to the tip of its bottom. This is used to calculate the age of the pregnancy from 6–13 weeks.

CVS: See **chorionic villus sampling**.

Cystic fibrosis: An inherited condition resulting in excessively thick mucous. It tends to clog the lungs and results in lung infections. Affected children used to die in their teens but now many live longer.

Cystic hygroma: Large fluid filled cysts in the soft tissues of the skin around the head and neck. This is seen in Turner syndrome and some other conditions.

Diagnostic test: A test which can determine accurately if a specific disease is present.

Diamniotic: When twins have their own separate bag of amniotic fluid surrounding each of them. Twins are diamniotic in all but very rare circumstances.

Diaphragmatic hernia: When there is a defect in the muscular layer between the chest and the abdominal cavities. As a result, some of the contents of the abdominal cavity ride up into the chest.

Dichorionic: Twins that have two separate placentas, The two placentas may be joined but there is no blood vessel communication between the two fetuses.

Dilatation and curettage: A surgical technique involving dilating (or enlarging the opening of) the cervix to remove the contents of the uterus. Also known as a D&C or a curette.

Dizygous: Non-identical twins who develop from two separate fertilized eggs, and are no more alike than brothers or sisters. See **monozygous**.

DNA (deoxyribonucleic acid): The chemical found inside a cell that carries the genetic instructions for making living organisms.

Dominant condition: People who carry one copy of the gene defect for a specific condition will develop the disease. A parent affected by the disease will have a 1 in 2 chance of passing it on to his or her children. An example is Huntington's disease.

Doppler: An ultrasound technique that shows the speed and direction of blood flowing in blood vessels. With color Doppler, blood flow is shown as blue or red in an ultrasound image. Pulsed Doppler produces a tracing of blood flow.

Down syndrome: A condition in which an individual carries three copies of chromosome 21 instead of the normal two copies. It results in severe intellectual handicap and commonly other physical abnormalities. Also called **trisomy 21.**

Duchenne muscular dystrophy: A condition that begins in early childhood and produces increasing muscular weakness. It usually results in death in early adulthood.

Ectopic pregnancy: A pregnancy that develops outside the uterine cavity, usually in a fallopian tube.

Edward syndrome: See **trisomy 18.**

Embryo: The conceptus early in pregnancy. The embryo technically becomes a fetus at 10 weeks, For convenience, 'fetus' is commonly used to include both the embryo and the fetus later in pregnancy.

Exomphalos: See **omphalocele.**

False negative: A normal test result, despite the person having the disease for which they are being tested.

False positive: An abnormal test result, which incorrectly suggests that an abnormality is present when it is not.

Fetal blood sampling: A sample of blood taken from the fetus by passing a fine needle through the skin of the pregnant woman into the uterus and then into a blood vessel, usually in the umbilical cord. Also called FBS and cordocentesis.

Fibroid: These are thickenings of muscle and fibrous tissue in the wall of uterus. Also called fibromyoma.

FISH (fluorescent in situ hybridization): A DNA technique that allows some chromosome abnormalities to be tested within 24–48 hours of an amniocentesis or CVS.

Folate: This is folic acid or vitamin B6. A shortage of folate has been shown to increase the chance of spina bifida.

Fragile X: The most common cause of inherited intellectual handicap— mild to severe in males and mild to moderate in females. It is caused by an abnormality in the X chromosome.

Gastroschisis: A defect in the abdominal wall where there is no covering over the bowel contents and they protrude into the amniotic cavity.

Gene: A small portion of a chromosome, composed of DNA, that is responsible for controlling a specific inherited characteristic of a person.

Genetic counselor: A person who provides counseling to people about genetic diseases. They are not medically trained, but are trained in counseling and in inherited diseases. It is available through genetics units, which are usually based in children's hospitals.

Genetic disease: A disease that is passed on from generation to generation through the genes.

Geneticist: A doctor specialising in genetic diseases.

Haemophilia: An inherited bleeding disorder caused by the blood lacking a protein involved in clotting.

Harelip: see **Cleft lip**.

Huntington's chorea: An inherited dominant condition causing severe body twitches and clumsiness plus intellectual deterioration after the age of 40.

Hydrocephalus: The accumulation of fluid in the chambers, or ventricles, of the brain. Also known as water on the brain.

Hydronephrosis: A blockage in the drainage of urine from the kidney that results in enlargement of the collecting system within the kidney.

Hydrops: Excessive accumulation of fluid in the tissues of the body.

Hypoplasia: Incomplete development of an organ, for example, a hypoplastic left heart is when the left side of the heart is underdeveloped.

Increased risk: The results of screening tests are usually given as increased risk or low risk. In prenatal testing, this most often refers to the risk of Down syndrome. Those with an increased risk are offered further testing. Most women with an increased risk of Down syndrome choose to have amniocentesis or CVS to obtain a definite result.

Intrauterine treatment: Treatment of the fetus, prior to birth.

Intravascular transfusion: A transfusion of blood into the circulation of the fetus, usually into a blood vessel in the umbilical cord. The most common reason for this is when the blood groups of the pregnant woman and fetus are incompatibile, such as in **Rhesus disease**.

Karyotype: A photograph of the chromosomes arranged in order to determine the chromosome number and structure of each.

Klinefelter syndrome: A syndrome affecting boys with an extra X chromosome, giving them a total of 47 chromosomes. Such boys are tall, they may have a mild reduction in intelligence, and frequently have specific learning problems. They are infertile.

Lethal abnormality: An abnormality that is so serious that death is expected either during pregnancy or shortly after birth. Examples include **anencephaly, hydrops** (if severe), a complete blockage of the fetal urine output (if untreated), **spina bifida** (if severe), **trisomy 13, trisomy 18,** and some dwarfism conditions.

Major abnormality: An abnormality of the fetus that is expected to cause significant disability, such as severe **hydrocephalus**, severe **hydronephrosis** and some types of congenital heart disease.

Marker chromosome: A small additional chromosome of unidentified origin in addition to the normal 46.

Markers (or 'soft' signs): Changes noted on ultrasound in the appearance of fetal physical structures. They cause no harm in themselves, but can sometimes be associated with a more serious condition. Many markers have been identified for Down syndrome, including neck swelling (nuchal oedema).

Maternal cell contamination: These are cells grown in the laboratory after amniocentesis or CVS that come from the pregnant woman rather than the fetus. Rarely they can cause difficulties in interpreting the findings.

Maternal serum alpha-fetoprotein: See **alpha-fetoprotein**.

Maternal serum screening: A test that indicates the risk of Down syndrome from a blood sample taken from the pregnant woman. Also called **serum screening, triple test** (if three different substances are tested) or **quadruple test** (if four are tested).

Minor abnormality: An abnormality that is not expected to result in any major problems for the baby after birth.

Miscarriage: See also **abortion** (spontaneous). A missed miscarriage is when the fetus dies sometime before the start of bleeding. A threatened miscarriage is any bleeding in early pregnancy. A miscarriage when the fetus cannot be seen is called a **blighted ovum**.

Monoamniotic: Identical twins that share a single amniotic sac. This very rare situation is a high-risk pregnancy, because the cords of the fetuses usually become entangled.

Monochorionic: Twins with a single placenta whose circulations mix in the placenta.

Monozygous twins: Identical twins, derived from a single fertilized egg.

Mosaicism: When an individual has different chromosome populations in different cells. 'True' mosaicism is when the fetus itself has different chromosome populations in different cells. Pseudo mosaicism is when the fetus has no abnormality and the apparent mosaicism occurred in the laboratory. Confined placental mosaicism is when the abnormal chromosomes are in a portion of the placenta but not in the fetus itself.

Negative result: A normal result, that is, a result that does not show an abnormality. A negative result should not be confused with a negative, or poor, outcome. See also **positive result.**

Neural tube defect (NTD): An abnormality of the nervous system involving the spine (**spina bifida**) or skull (**anencephaly** or encephalocele).

Nuchal translucency: The fluid layer beneath the skin at the back of the fetal neck. It is present in all fetuses at 10–13 weeks. If it is thicker than normal it may be called nuchal thickening or nuchal oedema. Measuring nuchal translucency is a screening test for **Down syndrome.**

Omphalocele: (also called exomphalos) A deficiency in the skin and muscle of the abdominal wall in which the contents are covered by a membrane.

Osteogenesis imperfecta: Brittle bones resulting in fractures after birth and sometimes before birth.

Parvo virus (or slap cheek virus): A mild infection common in schools. If a pregnant woman develops parvo virus early in her pregnancy, there is a risk of miscarriage. It can occasionally cause severe fetal anaemia.

Patau Syndrome: See **trisomy 13**.

Polymerase chain reaction (PCR): A DNA technique for testing for chromosome or gene defects.

Placenta praevia: When the placenta is implanted into the lower part of the uterus. This often results in bleeding, which may be severe, in the later stages of pregnancy. A delivery by caesarean section may be necessary.

Positive result: An abnormal result, that is, a result showing the fetus has the condition for which it is being tested. A positive result should not be confused with a positive, or good, outcome. See also **negative result**.

Pyelectasis: A small increase in the amount of fluid in the collecting system of the fetal kidney. It can be associated with kidney problems after birth, but these are usually not severe.

Quadruple test: Maternal serum screening is called the quadruple test if four substances in the pregnant woman's blood are analyzed.

Recessive: A condition that is harmless to individuals who carry only one copy of the gene. If both parents carry the gene defect, 1 in 4 of their children will develop the disease. The best known example of this is **cystic fibrosis**.

Rhesus disease: A blood group incompatibility between a pregnant woman (whose blood group is Rhesus negative) and her fetus (whose blood group is Rhesus positive). Rhesus disease is prevented by a blood product called anti-D, or Rhogam.

Rubella (German measles): A common childhood illness that can cause severe fetal abnormalities if caught by a pregnant woman. Now that schoolgirls are vaccinated, it has become less of a problem.

Screening test: A test done on large numbers of apparently healthy individuals, which aims to identify those at increased risk of a particular disorder. Most screening tests are not 100 per cent accurate. They have **false positive** and **false negative** results. See also **diagnostic test**.

Selective fetal reduction: A procedure in which one fetus in a multiple pregnancy, that is known to have an abnormality, is injected with a lethal substance.

Serum screening: See **maternal serum screening**.

Sex chromosome abnormality: An abnormality in the number or structure of one of the two sex chromosomes.

Sex-linked conditions: These are gene disorders that are only likely to affect the sons of women who are carriers. The woman herself has no symptoms, but each son has a 1 in 2 chance of being born with the disease. Examples are **haemophilia** and **Duchenne muscular dystrophy**.

Sonographer: An individual trained in the technique of carrying out ultrasound examinations. The sonographer is not medically trained.

Sonologist: A doctor who is trained to carry out ultrasound examinations.

Spina bifida: A defect in the vertebral column which often results in the nerves of the spinal cord protruding into the skin. It usually occurs low in the baby's back and causes varying degrees of paralysis of the legs, bladder, and bowel.

Syndrome: A combination of defects resulting in a distinct clinical picture.

Tay-Sachs disease: A recessive condition that is common in Ashkenazi Jews.

Termination of pregnancy: See **abortion**.

Thalassaemia: A recessive inherited condition resulting in severe anaemia that is common in people who originate from Mediterranean countries.

Translocation: A chromosome abnormality in which two chromosomes swap a portion of their genetic material.

Trimester: There are three trimesters of pregnancy; months 1,2 and 3 are the first trimester; months 4, 5, and 6 are the second trimester; and months 7, 8, and 9 are the third trimester.

Triple test: Serum screening may be called a triple test if three substances are analyzed in the pregnant woman's blood.

Triploidy: When a fetus receives three copies of each chromosome instead of the usual two. It then has 69 chromosomes in total. This is a very common cause of early miscarriage. Occasionally triploid fetuses can live until late in pregnancy, but have multiple abnormalities and severe growth delay.

Trisomy: An individual with an additional chromosome i.e. a total of 47 chromosomes.

Trisomy 13 (Patau syndrome): An individual with an additional chromosome 13. This results in severe intellectual impairment and many physical abnormalities. It usually results in death either before or immediately after birth.

Trisomy 18 (Edward syndrome): An individual with an additional chromosome 18. This usually causes the fetus to die during pregnancy or shortly after birth. A small percentage live longer but have profound intellectual incapacity and other physical problems.

Trisomy 21: See **Down syndrome**.

Turner syndrome (monosomy X): A female who has only one instead of the usual two X chromosomes.

Twin-to-twin transfusion: A twin pregnancy in which blood from the two fetuses mixes in the placenta, with more of the blood being transferred from one twin (the donor twin) to the other twin (the recipient twin).

Ultrasound scan: This involves high frequency sound waves being passed into the body and the reflected echoes being analyzed to build up a picture of the fetus in the uterus. It is painless and considered safe in pregnancy.

Villi: The microscopic finger-like structures that project out from the placenta toward the lining of the uterus.

Water on the brain: See **hydrocephalus**.

Contacts

Useful internet addresses

We suggest the internet or world-wide-web be used cautiously in searching for information about prenatal testing and fetal abnormality. Anybody can add whatever information they wish to the web. It is frequently inaccurate and makes no allowance for individual cases and the different outcomes related to the severity of conditions and the weeks of gestation. We encourage you to work with your doctor to obtain information, perhaps to locate appropriate web sites, and to seek further opinions if you wish. Below, however, are some addresses that may contain useful information.

<http://www.arc-uk.org/>   ARC is the only UK national charity which provides non-directive support and information to parents throughout the antenatal testing process. They help parents arrive at the most appropriate decision for them in the context of their family life.

<http://www.TheFetus.net>   The purpose of this site is to provide assistance to those who perform prenatal diagnosis and to the parents of fetuses possibly affected by problems.

<http://my.webmd.com/webmd_today/home/default>   WebMD provides health information, including during pregnancy and some discussion of prenatal testing, tools for managing your health, and support to those who seek information.

<http://www.nlm.nih.gov/medlineplus/pregnancy.html>   MedlinePlus provides good health information from the world's largest medical library, the National Library of Medicine. It provides authoratative and up to date information for health professionals and consumers.

<http://www.ncbi.nlm.nih.gov/entrez/query.fcgi>   PubMed, a service of the National Library of Medicine, includes over 15 million citations for biomedical articles back to the 1950s. These are from MEDLINE and

additional life science journals. PubMed includes links to many sites providing full text articles and other related resources.

<http://www.cdc.gov/health/womensmenu.htm> The Centers for Disease Control and Prevention (CDC) is a leading US government agency for protecting the health and safety of people by providing credible information to enhance health decisions.

<http://www.ob-ultrasound.net/> Information about obstetric ultrasound, including other references.

<http://www.melbuswomen.com.au> The site of one of the authors of this book. It contains, in summary form, the information on prenatal tests that is presented in more detail in this book.

LIBRARY, UNIVERSITY OF CHESTER

Index

Note: Page numbers in **bold** indicate tables and figures.